Preparing for
ICD-10-CM:
Make the Transition Manageable

Deborah J. Grider, CPC, CPC-H, CCS-P, CCP

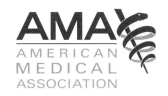

AMA
AMERICAN
MEDICAL
ASSOCIATION

Executive Vice President, Chief Executive Officer: Michael D. Maves, MD, MBA
Chief Operating Officer: Bernard L. Hengesbaugh
Senior Vice President, Publishing and Business Services: Robert A. Musacchio, PhD
Vice President and General Manager, Publishing: Frank J. Krause
Vice President, Business Operations: Vanessa Hayden
Publisher, Physician Practice Solutions: Jay T. Ahlman
Senior Acquisitions Editor: Elise Schumacher
Manager, Book and Product Development and Production: Nancy C. Baker
Senior Developmental Editor: Lisa Chin-Johnson
Director, Business Marketing and Communication: Pam Palmersheim
Director, Sales and Strategic Partnerships: J. D. Kinney
Production Manager: Rosalyn Carlton
Senior Print Production Specialist: Ronnie Summers
Production Specialist: Mary Ann Albanese
Marketing Manager: Leigh Adams

The authors, editors, and publisher of this work have checked with sources believed to be reliable in their efforts to confirm the accuracy and completeness of the information presented herein and that the information is in accordance with the standard practices accepted at the time of publication. However, neither the authors nor the publisher nor any party involved in the creation and publication of this work warrant that the information is in every respect accurate and complete, and they are not responsible for any errors or omissions or for any consequences from application of the information in this book.

Additional copies of this book may be ordered by calling 800 621-8335 or from the secure AMA web site at www.amabookstore.com. Refer to product number OP602608.

ISBN 978-1-57947-866-7

BP30:09-P-044:10/09

Library of Congress Cataloging-in-Publication Data
Grider, Deborah J.
     Preparing for ICD-10-CM : make the transition manageable / Deborah J. Grider.
          p. ; cm.
     Includes index.
     Summary: "This book provides a history of ICD-10-CM, identifies differences between coding diagnoses with ICD-9-CM versus ICD-10-CM, and provides guidance on how physicians and medical practices can begin planning for implementation of ICD-10-CM"—Provided by publisher.
     ISBN 978-1-57947-866-7
   1. Nosology—Code numbers. 2. International classification of diseases, 10th revision, clinical modification. I. American Medical Association. II. International classification of diseases, 10th revision, clinical modification. III. Title.
     [DNLM: 1. International classification of diseases, 10th revision, clinical modification. 2. Disease—classification. 3. Diagnosis. 4. Information Systems. WB 15 G847p 2010]
          RB115.G7495 2010
          616.001'48—dc22
     2009014254

Table of Contents

Chapter 3   Migration to ICD-10-CM   23

Chapter 4   Implementation of ICD-10-CM for Physicians and Staff   41

Preface

Diagnosis coding is the transformation of narrative descriptions of diseases, injuries, and medical procedures into numeric or alphanumeric designations that are grouped together into manageable categories. Accurate diagnosis coding is critical because it is the basis for obtaining medical data for the following:

- Reporting and trending vital health statistics in the United States and worldwide
- Evaluating medical processes and outcomes
- Reporting data to governmental and private organizations charged with overseeing the quality and cost effectiveness of care
- Identifying public health issues and concerns
- Identifying ways to improve the safety and quality of care
- Evaluating medical necessity when adjudicating health care claims.

The Current Coding System: ICD-9-CM

ICD-9-CM stands for *International Classification of Diseases, Ninth Revision, Clinical Modification*, which is the US version of ICD-9 developed by the World Health Organization (WHO). ICD-9-CM is divided into three volumes: Volumes 1 and 2 relate to diagnoses classification, and Volume 3 relates to the inpatient procedure classification.

ICD-9-CM has become obsolete because it was developed in the early 1970s. It has been in use since 1979. Many of the clinical and procedural concepts in ICD-9-CM are no longer able to meet today's demanding health care data needs, and, like technology and outdated software and equipment that are no longer supported by the developer, ICD-9 is no longer supported by WHO and, therefore, cannot be significantly modified to meet current and future needs.

ICD-10 is the tenth revision of the classification system and includes a code set for diagnoses ("CM") and a code set for procedures ("PCS"). ICD-10-CM will provide improved data to meet the demand of the increasingly global and electronic health care environment. Studies indicate that the United States needs to adopt and implement ICD-10-CM in the near future as a national clinical coding system in order to improve the quality of patient care and health data. ICD-9-CM is obsolete. Developed nearly 30 years ago, it cannot accurately describe the diagnoses and inpatient procedures of care delivered today.

The ways in which coded data are being used today go well beyond the purposes for which ICD-9-CM was designed back in the 1970s. Significant advances in the understanding of disease and treatment have been made within the last 30 years. ICD-9-CM is not equipped to expand in the way technology is moving. ICD-10-CM provides a significant opportunity to improve the capture of information about the increasingly complex delivery of health care. ICD-10-CM will provide improved data for improved public health, will support quality of care and patient safety, and will provide more complete and accurate data in support of medical necessity and, in turn, reimbursement.

Another advantage of ICD-10-CM is that it is better suited for technology and use with the electronic health record (EHR) and electronic medical record (EMR) than ICD-9-CM is. More robust mapping from the Systematized Nomenclature of Medicine—Clinical Terms (SNOMED-CT) will be realized with ICD-10-CM, which will improve the value of clinical data to facilitate the retrieval of coded data at the desired level of detail depending on the purpose for which the data will be used.

Many other countries have adopted ICD-10 and are using this system today. Replacing ICD-9-CM with ICD-10-CM is necessary in order to maintain clinical data comparability with the rest of the world. It has become increasingly difficult to share disease and mortality data with an outdated system.

The United States has been using ICD-10 since 1999 for mortality reporting only. ICD-10-CM implementation is necessary in order to maintain comparability between mortality and morbidity data with the world. This book will provide guidance in identifying key points and strategies that an organization should implement when making the transition from ICD-9-CM to ICD-10-CM. The task will not be easy but, with the proper information, guidance, preparation, and training, the transition can be smoother.

Objectives of This Book

The objectives of *Preparing for ICD-10-CM: Make the Transition Manageable* are as follows:

- Provide information about the history and migration to ICD-10-CM and its importance
- Identify the differences between coding diagnoses with ICD-9-CM versus ICD-10-CM
- Provide guidance on how physicians and medical practices can begin planning for implementation of ICD-10-CM
- Review chapters, tables, and guidelines of ICD-10-CM
- Minimize the impact of change for the physician practice.

Very little time remains to plan for this change in coding diagnoses. All staff members, physicians, other clinical staff members, managers, administrators, and coders must learn about ICD-10-CM and how to use it appropriately in order for it to be successfully implemented throughout the health care industry.

Foreword

Change in the medical environment is imminent. After 30 years, the nation's physicians will be required to report diagnostic codes based on the ICD-10 code set. The American Medical Association (AMA) understands the need to work with up-to-date health care standards and code sets, and in light of such changes it has published *Preparing for ICD-10-CM: Make the Transition Manageable*. The AMA realizes that the move to ICD-10 will be a costly and time-consuming endeavor for physicians. We are deeply concerned about the strain this will place on physicians, especially since the transition to ICD-10 comes in the midst of other significant health technology changes for physician practices, as well as a weakened economy. The Medicare Physician Quality Reporting Initiative, the electronic program established under the Medicare Improvements for Patients and Providers Act of 2008, and an electronic heath record system program established in the newly enacted American Recovery and Reinvestment Act of 2009 are among the many other changes physicians will be contending with, and each will require additional resources to implement. But through the AMA's publishing efforts, we hope to ease the transition to ICD-10-CM as much as possible by providing information needed to begin the change.

The Department of Health and Human Services (HHS) as well as several other health care industry stakeholders were keen on moving to ICD-10; however, given the time and resources physicians will need to expend in order to adopt ICD-10 codes, the AMA advocated vigorously against a speedy adoption time frame. During the summer of 2008, HHS initiated the regulatory process to move forward with the adoption of ICD-10-CM and ICD-10-PCS. The initial proposed date for compliance was October 1, 2011. The AMA, along with more than 100 physician state and specialty societies, expressed deep concerns in comments to HHS on the aggressive deadline to complete this complex transition. The final rule replacing ICD-9-CM with ICD-10-CM and ICD-10-PCS was published by HHS on January 16, 2009, and established a compliance date of October 1, 2013. Physician practices will need extensive time and resources to modify workflows and business practices to ensure that ICD-10 is appropriately and correctly integrated into their day-to-day business and clinical operations.

Before physician practices can even begin the large undertaking of implementing ICD-10, they need to first upgrade their administrative systems to replace the current HIPAA electronic transaction standard, version 4010, with version 5010. This upgrade must take place before the implementation of ICD-10 because version 4010 of the transactions does not accommodate the new structure and format of the ICD-10 codes. The compliance date for this implementation is January 1, 2012. Practices will need time to complete testing of and migration to the updated HIPAA electronic transactions with their trading partners in order to avoid significant disruptions to their practice, patient care, and claims payments.

The AMA has begun preparing an outreach plan and materials to support physicians as they embark on this significant change to their business and clinical processes. We will continue to advocate and provide resources related to the implementation of ICD-10 as we help doctors help patients. Look for more information on ICD-10 on our web site at www.ama-assn.org.

Michael D. Maves, MD, MBA
Executive Vice President, CEO

About the Author

Deborah J. Grider is a Certified Professional Coder-Instructor (CPC-I), a Certified Professional Coder Payer (CPC-P), a Certified OB/GYN Specialty Coder (COBGC), a Certified E/M Coder (CEMC), and a Certified Dermatology Specialty Coder (CEMC). Her background includes many years of practical experience in reimbursement issues, procedural and diagnostic coding, and medical practice management.

Ms Grider teaches and consults with private practices, physician networks, and hospital-based educational programs. Under a federal retraining grant, she helped develop and implement a Medical Assisting Program for Methodist Hospital of Indiana. Ms Grider is a national speaker conducting many seminars and workshops throughout the year on coding and reimbursement issues and teaches several insurance courses, including the Professional Medical Coder Curriculum, of which she is an approved instructor by the AAPC. Ms Grider also developed a Medical Coding Certificate Program for Clarian Health Partners, Inc, and Martin University in Indianapolis, Indiana.

Ms Grider is a national speaker for the AAPC as well as for other nationally known organizations. She is a former national advisory board member for the American Academy of Professional Coders. Prior to joining the AAPC in 2009, Ms Grider was President of Medical Professionals, Inc, for 15 years and provided consulting services to physician practices nationwide. Ms Grider also worked as a billing manager for 6 years, and a practice manager in a specialty practice for 12 years. As vice president of Strategic Development for the American Academy of Professional Coders, Ms Grider continues to provide educational services to medical groups, physician practices, and large hospital organizations and provides coding training education to numerous health care organizations and state medical societies.

Her professional affiliations include the AAPC; the Central Indiana Chapter of the AAPC of which she was the founder and president from 1996-1999 and 2001–2004; AAPC National Advisory Board Member 2002–2009; Chairman of the American Medical Association Liason Committee; member of AHIMA; corporate sponsor for the Indiana Medical Group Management Association; member of the National Association of Female Executives (NAFE); and a member of the Indianapolis Chamber of Commerce. She is in charge of ICD-10 training curriculum development for the American Academy of Professional Coders and is the past president of the American Academy of Professional Coders National Advisory Board.

Ms Grider was awarded her bachelor's degree in business administration from Indiana University.

CHAPTER 1

Introduction to ICD-10-CM

OBJECTIVES

- Understand the purpose of the International Classification of Diseases, Tenth Revision, Clinical Modification (ICD-10-CM)
- Understand the changes in our diagnosis coding system of the future
- Understand the need for changing our current diagnosis coding system
- Review the regulatory process involved with updating the codes

Introduction to ICD

ICD stands for the International Statistical Classification of Diseases and Health Related Problems. ICD was originally developed to classify mortality by promoting international comparability in the collection, processing, classification, and presentation of mortality statistics as well as providing a format for reporting causes of death on death certificates. In addition to being the international standard for recording causes of death, ICD was later expanded to classify morbidity. Both the International Classification of Diseases, Ninth Revision, Clinical Modification (ICD-9-CM) and ICD-10-CM have been clinically modified for use in the United States. *ICD-9* and *ICD-10* are the abbreviated terms to refer to the volumes and codes sets that make up each overall code set.

ICD-10 involves two components: (1) ICD-10-CM and (2) ICD-10-PCS (*PCS* stands for procedural coding system). ICD-9-CM has three volumes. Volumes 1 and 2 are used to report diagnosis codes, such as on health care claim forms to support medical necessity for services provided to patients. Volume 3 is for reporting inpatient hospital procedures. In the outpatient setting, Current Procedural Terminology and the Healthcare Common Procedure Coding System are used to report procedures and services.

ICD-10-CM currently is used to code and classify mortality data from death certificates, having replaced ICD-9-CM for this purpose as of January 1, 1999. However, ICD-9-CM remains the code set in use in the United States for morbidity. The discussion in this book will focus on the pending move from ICD-9-CM to ICD-10-CM for reporting morbidity.

In the United States, ICD-9-CM is the code set adopted for use under the Health Insurance Portability and Accountability Act (HIPAA) for reporting morbidities. The US Department of Health and Human Services (HHS) has proposed adopting ICD-10-CM as the new code set for reporting morbidities. The final rule naming the replacement of ICD-9-CM with ICD-10-CM was published in the *Federal Register* on January 16, 2009. The final rule established the requirement to use only ICD-10-CM for encounters or discharges on or after October 1, 2013.

Use of the new code set will provide a significant opportunity to improve the capture of information within our increasingly complex health care delivery system. ICD-10-CM promises to provide an enormous opportunity for documentation improvement for health records. More documentation in the medical record might be necessary to support reporting the specificity required using ICD-10-CM for diagnosis coding. ICD-10 will provide greater coding specificity to support accurate payment for hospitals, physicians, health plans, and others within the health system.

Health care providers and health plans need to begin preparation for the transition from ICD-9-CM to ICD-10-CM now. Key areas that need to be considered initially include staffing, vendor software, computer technology issues, clinical systems, information management, and the impact on cash flow.

What Is ICD-10?

When ICD-10 is implemented, ICD-10-CM will replace ICD-9-CM Volumes 1 and 2 for reporting diagnoses, and ICD-10-PCS will replace ICD-9-CM Volume 3 for reporting hospital inpatient procedures. ICD-10-PCS will not replace Current Procedural Terminology or the Healthcare Common Procedure Coding System for reporting procedures in outpatient settings.

ICD-10-CM codes are used by health care providers in both inpatient and outpatient settings to report diagnoses to support medical necessity for services provided. Several countries including the United States have developed clinical modifications to ICD for the purposes of meeting their own health care needs when reporting morbidities.

Diagnosis coding is the language of reporting why a service was medically necessary for patient care. Health plans require accurate reporting of diagnosis coding to explain why a service was provided to the patient.

ICD-10-CM, with its alphanumeric structure, will provide more specific information, expand injury coding, and provide a more descriptive clinical picture of the patient than does ICD-9-CM. ICD-10-CM contains more codes and categories that allow for more specific and accurate representation of current and future medical diagnoses and procedures.

Understanding Who Maintains the ICD-10 Code Set

In order to understand the ICD-10 code sets, one must understand the various agencies involved in the ICD-10 maintenance process.

ICD-10-PCS

ICD-10-PCS was developed as a replacement for ICD-9-CM Volume 3. This version of ICD, in use since January 1979, originated in the International Classification of Procedures in Medicine (ICPM). The ICPM was published by the World Health Organization (WHO) in 1978 for trial purposes. The classification consisted of nine chapters, with the first digit of the three-digit or four-digit code denoting the chapter number. ICD-10-PCS was developed by the 3M Corporation as a replacement for ICD-9-CM Volume 3. The Centers for Medicare & Medicaid Services (CMS) is responsible for the maintenance of ICD-10-CM Volume 3 and ICD-10-PCS.

World Health Organization (WHO)

WHO is the international agency that maintains an international nomenclature of mortality and morbidity statistics, including causes of death, and public health reporting. The original intent of ICD-10, which was adopted in 1994, was as a statistical tool for tracking morbidity and mortality data. Since then, ICD-10 has become the international standard diagnostic classification for many health management purposes. The WHO owns and has published the classification in a three-volume set and is responsible for the development of the adaptation of ICD-10 for use in the United States.

The National Center for Health Statistics

The National Center for Health Statistics (NCHS) is the federal agency within the Centers for Disease Control and Prevention responsible for the development and clinical modification of ICD-10-CM in the United States. The NCHS, with guidance from CMS, revises ICD-9-CM.

Some other countries have developed a clinical modification to meet their own diagnoses reporting needs. For example, Canada has modified ICD-10 and calls it ICD-10-CA, whereas Australia has its own modification called ICD-10-AU.

The Need for Change

Many argue that the ICD-9-CM system has outgrown its intended level of specificity, which has an impact on the ability to compare data efficiently and precisely for research, clinical support, and appropriate reimbursement. ICD-9-CM has been in use since 1979 and no longer reflects advances in medical treatment. Many argue that an expandable system is needed. Terminologies and classifications from the 1970s no longer fit with the 21st century health care system, because numerous conditions and procedures are outdated and inconsistent with current medical knowledge and application. New advances in medicine and medical technology and the growing need for quality data cannot be accommodated.

The need to replace ICD-9-CM was identified in 1993, and steps were taken by the National Committee on Vital and Health Statistics (NCVHS)—a body that advises HHS on HIPAA matters—NCHS, and CMS to develop a plan for migration to ICD-10 for morbidity and mortality coding. ICD-10 use for mortality coding in the United States was initiated in 1999. Although many countries are now using variations of ICD-10, the United States continues with the now-unsupported ICD-9-CM (WHO now exclusively supports ICD-10). This leads to difficulties in comparing US data with that of the rest of the global community.

The most significant delay in converting to ICD-10-CM is the tremendous cost involved. According to a RAND Corporation study, the cost is estimated to be between $425 million and $1.15 billion in onetime costs for training and system changes for providers, health plans, hospitals, and vendors and between $5 and $40 million in lost productivity. Another significant reason for the delay is that transaction formats need to have the correct field length to send into clearinghouses. For example, the physician format defined by CMS1500 has five positions for the diagnosis field. The layout must be converted from version 4010 to version 5010 to allow for the additional digits. Currently, version 4010/4010A1 of the Accredited Standards Committee X12 group cannot accommodate the much larger ICD-10 code sets. The 5010 final rule mandates conversion to Version 5010 on January 1, 2012, prior to ICD-10 implementation. HIPAA gave HHS the responsibility for designating a standard code set with which to describe diagnoses and procedures. At the time, ICD-10 was not yet ready to be mandated, and so ICD-9-CM was chosen instead. One drawback was that ICD-10-CM did not have the capability to report procedures as with ICD-9-CM Volume 3. In addition, a cost-benefit analysis needed to be performed before ICD-10 could be adopted.

ICD-9-CM lacks specificity and detail for reporting diagnoses, no longer reflects current knowledge of disease processes, and hampers the ability to compare costs and outcomes of different medical technologies. In addition, ICD-9-CM does not meet the need for new services and technology that must be acknowledged in CMS payment systems according to the Benefits Improvement and Protection Act of 2000, which modifies Medicare's payment rates for many services and adds coverage of certain preventive and therapeutic services. It also makes changes to both Medicaid and the State Children's Health Insurance Program.

Significant costs are incurred by continued use of severely outdated and limited coding systems. For example, failure of our coding systems to keep pace with medical advances results in the use of vague or incorrect codes, which in the situation of claims processing, often requires excessive reliance on supporting paper documentation (ie, attachments or copies of the health record).

According to the May 4, 2001, *Federal Register*, the ICD-9-CM procedure coding system is limited to a maximum of 10,000 codes, most of which are already assigned. ICD-9-CM has limitations with a four-digit structure that does not allow for much change. In 1993, NCVHS indicated to HHS that ICD-9-CM was running out of code numbers. Deficiencies in ICD-9-CM include:

- insufficient structure for reporting new technology;
- duplicate codes and codes that overlap;
- outdated terminology;
- insufficient specificity and detail; and
- lack of codes for certain types of conditions or services.

In the HHS proposed rule for electronic transactions and code sets under HIPAA, it was noted that ICD-9-CM has limited availability to accommodate new procedures and diagnoses and lacks the precision needed for biosurveillance and pay-for-performance. In addition, ICD-9-CM lacks specificity and detail, uses terminology inconsistently, cannot capture new technology, and will eventually run out of space, especially in ICD-9-CM Volume 3. ICD-9-CM has become outdated and obsolete, and the need for a diagnosis coding source has gone beyond the original scope of the document as it was adopted.

Providers are consistently required to use multiple coding systems to meet the needs of multiple health plans for reimbursement, research, profiling, outcomes measurement, and case-mix management. Some of the pertinent reasons we use coding data today are to:

- identify fraudulent practices;
- support medical necessity;
- research and support clinical trials;
- set health policy;
- process claims for reimbursement; and
- measure quality and efficacy of care.

Progress toward adoption of ICD-10 began well over a decade ago. Extensive work and dedication have gone into developing and evaluating this system as a replacement for ICD-9. Although there is significant support for this, many health care organizations believe that the cost of moving to ICD-10 will be enormous and that the move is unnecessary. Physicians and other health care professionals are facing a staggering number of technological requirements, including multiple overlapping federal mandates that place significant financial and operational burdens on practices, especially smaller ones.

Overview of the ICD-10-CM Coding System

ICD-10-CM was developed after a thorough evaluation, which included input from a technical advisory panel and consultation with physician groups, clinical coders, and relevant organizations to ensure accuracy and consistency in coding diagnoses. Some improvements with this clinical modification include:

- addition of information relevant to ambulatory and managed care encounters;
- creation of combination codes for diagnosis and symptoms, which will reduce the number of diagnosis codes required to describe a specific condition;
- expanded injury codes to include code extensions for injuries and external causes of injury;
- additional pregnancy trimester information;
- addition of up to seven characters;
- addition of common four-digit and five-digit subclassifications;
- laterality;
- expanded alcohol and substance abuse codes;
- expanded postoperative complication codes; and
- greater specificity in code assignment.

ICD-10-CM will dramatically affect the way we report diagnoses in the United States. The ICD code set has been revised periodically to incorporate changes in the medical field. ICD-10 differs from ICD-9 in a number of respects, although the overall content is similar.

- ICD-10 is printed in a three-volume set, whereas ICD-9 is a two-volume set.
- ICD-10 has alphanumeric categories rather than just numeric categories.
- Some chapters have been rearranged.
- Some titles have changed.
- Conditions have been regrouped.
- ICD-10 has almost twice as many categories as ICD-9 has.
- Minor changes have been made in the coding rules for mortality.

ICD-10 consists of the following:

- Tabular lists containing cause-of-death titles and codes (Volume 1)
- Inclusion and exclusion terms for cause-of-death titles (Volume 1)
- An alphabetical index to diseases and nature of injury
- External causes of injury
- Table of drugs and chemicals (Volume 3)
- Description, guidelines, and coding rules (Volume 2).

The process of converting from ICD-9-CM to ICD-10-CM affects many aspects of the mortality data system, including revision of instruction manuals and medical software.

Regulatory Process

While taking into account the diversity of input and lack of industry-wide consensus, NCVHS concluded that it is in the best interest of the country as a whole to adopt ICD-10 as the standard for national implementation as the replacement for current uses of ICD-9. As a result, NCVHS recommended that HHS initiate the regulatory process for the adoption of ICD-10.

The final rule for ICD-10 was published January 16, 2009, in the *Federal Register*. It modifies the standard medical data code sets for coding diagnoses and inpatient hospital procedures by adopting the ICD-10-CM for diagnosis coding, which includes the Official ICD-10-CM Guidelines for Coding and Reporting maintained and distributed by HHS and ICD-10-PCS for inpatient hospital procedure coding, including the Official ICD-10-PCS Guidelines for Coding and Reporting. These new codes sets, effective October 1, 2013, replace ICD-9-CM Volumes 1, 2, and 3, including the Official ICD-9-CM Guidelines for Coding and Reporting. The new book, however, will not address ICD-10-PCS.

As of October 1, 2013, all discharges and services must be coded using ICD-10. According to the ICD-10 final rule published January 16, 2009, ". . . for the period around October 1, 2013, the usual coding rule for inpatient services will apply: the code in use on the date of discharge not the date of admission will be the one employed; therefore, if a patient is discharged on or after October 1, 2013, ICD-10 must be used."

The proposed rule had called for a 2011 implementation date, but because of significant concerns by many health care organizations and medical societies that this was too aggressive, the date was pushed back to 2013 to allow for more time to prepare for the transition. The new date gives providers now using the ICD-9 code set an additional two years to prepare for compliance, which experts are contending will be costly and time consuming.

Because the current version of HIPAA standards, 4010, does not accommodate use of the ICD-10 codes, HHS also published on January 16, 2009, a final rule naming an updated version of the X12 transactions (version 5010) and an updated version of the National Council for Prescription Drug Programs standard (version D.0) for electronic, pharmacy-related transactions previously adopted under HIPAA. The final rule also names a standard transaction for Medicaid pharmacy subrogation. HHS extended the deadline for complying with the updated transactions by 21 months from the date set in the proposed rule, to January 1, 2012. Small health plans have an additional year to meet the compliance deadline for the new pharmacy subrogation transaction.

Summary

Now is the time to begin the vital preparation of ICD-10-CM in medical practice. Planning and preparation for this complex coding system must occur prior to implementation. Chapter 5 will provide an in-depth overview of necessary preparation along with timelines for accomplishing goals. It is important to remember that, without appropriate preparation, this change could affect a practice's operating efficiency and its revenue.

The current ICD-10-CM codes, including mapping to ICD-9-CM, Volumes 1 and 2, are further discussed in Chapter 9, are available on the CMS Web site at www.cms.hhs.gov/ICD10. Physicians and staff members are encouraged to review the coding structure, guidelines, and information related to ICD-10-CM and begin preparing for the transition now.

Resources

National Center for Health Statistics, International Classification of Diseases, Tenth Revision, Clinical Modification (ICD-10-CM). *About the International Classification of Diseases, Tenth Revision, Clinical Modification ICD-10-CM.* Available online at www.cdc.gov/nchs/about/otheract/icd9/ icd10cm.htm (accessed March 18, 2009).

National Center for Health Statistics. International Classification of Diseases, Ninth Revision, Clinical Modification (ICD-9-CM). Available online at www.cdc.gov/nchs/about/otheract/icd9/abticd9.htm (accessed March 18, 2009).

Current Procedural Terminology. Available online at www.cms.hhs.gov/ medhcpcsgeninfo/01_overview.asp (accessed March 18, 2009).

Healthcare Common Procedure Coding System. Available online at www.cms.hhs.gov/medhcpcsgeninfo/01_overview.asp (accessed March 18, 2009).

Health Insurance Portability and Accountability Act of 1996, 104th Cong, Pub L No. 104-191. Available online at www.cms.hhs.gov/HIPAAGenInfo/ Downloads/HIPAALaw.pdf (accessed March 18, 2009).

Federal Register. Vol. 74, No. 11. January 16, 2009. Rules and Regulations. ICD-10 Final Rule. Available online at edocket.access.gpo.gov/2009/pdf/ E9-743.pdf (accessed March 18, 2009).

World Health Organization. *International Classification of Procedures in Medicine.* Geneva, Switzerland: World Health Organization; 1978.

Centers for Medicare & Medicaid Services, 2008. *ICD-10-CM, July 2007 release.* Available online at www.cms.hhs.gov/ICD10 (accessed March 18, 2009).

American Hospital Association. *NCVHS Committee recommendation for I-10.* Available online at www.ahacentraloffice.org/ahacentraloffice/html/ icd10resources.html (accessed March 18, 2009).

September 2005 joint AdvaMed, AHA and Federation of American Hospitals letter in support of ICD-10 implementation. Available online at www.ahacentraloffice.org/ahacentraloffice/images/ICD-10 McClellanJGLogo.pdf (accessed March 18, 2009).

Library of Congress, US Senate bill 628. Introduced March 18, 2009. http://thomas.loc.gov/.

Lumpkin, J. *Letter to Tommy Thompson on ICD-10, November 5, 2003.* Available online at www.ncvhs.hhs.gov/031105lt.htm (accessed March 18, 2009).

American Health Information Management Association. *Why ICD-9 has to be replaced.* Available online at www.ahima.org/icd10/icd9.asp (accessed March 18, 2009).

Benefits Improvement and Protection Act of 2000. Available online at www.ncvhs.hhs.gov/020409p1.htm (accessed March 18, 2009).

Department of Health and Human Services. Final Rule, 5010. *Federal Register,* January 16, 2009. Available online at http://edocket.access.gpo.gov/2009/ pdf/E9-740.pdf (accessed March 18, 2009).

Department of Health and Human Services. Final Rule, ICD-10-CM. *Federal Register,* January 16, 2009. Available online at http://edocket.access.gpo. gov/2009/pdf/E9-743.pdf (accessed March 18, 2009).

End-of-Chapter Questions

1 ICD-10-CM will have up to _____ character extensions.

2 *WHO* stands for _____ _____ _____.

3 ICD-10-CM is currently used in the United States for

_____.

4 The ICD-10-CM format is:
   a. numeric.
   b. alphanumeric.
   c. alphabetical.

5 ICD-10-CM is published in a _____ volume set.

CHAPTER 2

Development of Clinical Modifications to the International Classification of Diseases

OBJECTIVES

- Understand the history of the International Classification of Diseases (ICD)
- Understand the background of ICD-10-CM development
- Review the rationale for change

Brief History and Background

The ICD began in the early 1800s, based on John Graunt's earlier work, *Natural and Political Observations Made Upon the Bills of Mortality* (1662). By 1937, this demographic method of tracking information had evolved into the International List of Causes of Death. The World Health Organization (WHO) published a statistical listing in 1948 that could be used to track both morbidity and mortality. Years later, the International Conference for the Ninth Revision of the International Classification of Diseases was convened by the WHO in Geneva in 1975. At this conference, the governing bodies were interested in using ICD for tracking mortality statistics. However, some subject areas in the WHO classification were inappropriately arranged, and more detail was needed to adapt the classification and make it more relevant.

This conference also made recommendations on a number of related technical subjects, and the following changes were made.

- Coding rules for mortality were amended slightly.
- Rules for the selection of a single cause for tabulation of morbidity were introduced.
- Definitions and recommendations for statistics in the field of perinatal mortality were amended and extended.
- Use of a certificate of causes of perinatal death was recommended.

In 1977, the National Center for Health Statistics (NCHS) developed a clinical modification for use in coding and reporting. The clinical modification of ICD-9 (ICD-9-CM, Volumes 1 and 2), which is still used today for reporting morbidities, was adopted for use in the United States in 1979. When ICD-9-CM was published, the NCHS decided to modify it to gather more clinical information to capture not only morbidity statistics in the United States but to capture mortality statistics as well.

In addition to its use in identifying mortality and morbidity, ICD-9-CM was adopted to classify diseases and health conditions for health care claims for hospitals, physicians, and other health care providers and facilities. ICD-9-CM is used to report not only diagnoses to facilitate payment of health services but also to evaluate utilization patterns, predict health care trends, analyze health care costs, research the quality of health care, and plan for future health care requirements.

ICD-9-CM also includes alternative methods of classifying diagnostic statements, in addition to information about manifestation of diseases related to organ or site and classifying the underlying disease. This system is known as the dagger and asterisk system and is retained in the Tenth Revision of ICD. Technical innovations were included in ICD-9-CM to increase the flexibility for worldwide use. The clinical modification added detail at the fourth- and fifth-digit subdivisions. This modification was designed to provide greater flexibility in many situations.

In the late 1970s, the United States also developed Volume 3 of ICD-9-CM to identify inpatient hospital procedures to use with Volumes 1 and 2. Volume 3 has been used since 1979 to report procedures performed in the hospital for hospital claims and statistics.

In 1983, the inpatient prospective payment system was adopted, and ICD-9-CM Volumes 1, 2, and 3 were used for assigning cases to the diagnosis-related groups. As a result of the advances in medicine since ICD-9-CM was implemented, the system must be updated and revised periodically. An annual updating process was established by the ICD-9-CM Coordination and Maintenance Committee to update ICD-9-CM on an annual basis. This committee was created as a forum for proposals to update ICD-9-CM. One representative from the NCHS and one from the Centers for Medicare & Medicaid Services (CMS) co-chair the committee meetings. Responsibility for maintenance of the ICD-9-CM is divided between the two agencies, with classification of diagnoses (Volumes 1 and 2) by NCHS and classification of procedures (Volume 3) by CMS.

Although the ICD-9-CM Coordination and Maintenance Committee is a federal committee, suggestions for modifications come from both the public and private sectors. When ICD-10-CM implementation occurs in 2013, the ICD-9-CM Coordination and Maintenance Committee will be renamed the ICD-10 Coordination and Maintenance Committee.

In 1988, Congress passed the Medicare Catastrophic Coverage Act, which required the use of ICD-9-CM codes for processing Medicare claims. Many commercial and other third-party payers followed Medicare's lead and adopted ICD-9-CM as the standard for reporting diagnoses to support medical necessity.

In 1993, ICD-10 was first released by the WHO. The NCHS first awarded a contract to the Center for Health Policy Studies to evaluate ICD-10 for use for morbidity in the United States. A technical advisory panel developed a prototype of ICD-10-CM in 1994. It was recommended, on the basis of the panel's findings, that the NCHS proceed with implementation of ICD-10-CM with revisions. Further work on ICD-10-CM was performed by the NCHS along with review of proposals from the ICD-9-CM Coordination and Maintenance Committee and input from medical and surgical specialty groups.

The Administrative Simplification provisions of the Health Insurance Portability and Accountability Act of 1996 (HIPAA) required the Department of Health and Human Services (HHS) to establish national standards for electronic health care transactions, code sets, and national identifiers for providers, health plans, and employers. It also addressed the security and privacy of health data. Industry use of these standards is aimed at greater health care system efficiency and effectiveness through improved use of standard electronic data interchange.

Under HIPAA, a code set is any set of codes used for encoding data elements, such as tables of terms, medical concepts, medical diagnosis codes, or medical procedure codes. Medical data code sets used in the health care industry include coding systems for diseases, impairments, other health-related problems, and their manifestations; causes of injury, disease, impairment, or other health-related problems; actions taken to prevent, diagnose, treat, or manage diseases, injuries, and impairments; and any substances, equipment, supplies, or other items used to perform these actions. Code sets for medical data are required data elements in the electronic administrative and financial health care transaction standards adopted under HIPAA for diagnoses, procedures, and drugs.

HIPAA has identified 10 standard transactions for electronic data interchange for the transmission of health care data. Claims and encounter information, payment and remittance advice, and claims status and inquiry are several of the standard transactions. Code sets are the codes used to identify specific diagnosis and clinical procedures on claims and encounter forms. Examples of code sets for procedures, diagnoses, and drugs with which providers are familiar include the Healthcare Common Procedures Coding System, Current Procedural Terminology, ICD-9, and National Drug Codes.

ICD-9-CM is used today not only for disease classification. It is the standard for payment justification and supporting medical necessity for a procedure or service provided to a patient in a health care setting. It has become our core classification system to code claims for commercial and government health insurance reimbursement.

With the release of ICD-10 Volume 1 in 1992 by the WHO, the United States was granted permission to develop an adaptation of ICD-10, which is referred to as ICD-10-CM (clinical modification) for government purposes.

Development of ICD-10-CM

The draft of ICD-10-CM, along with a preliminary crosswalk between ICD-9-CM and ICD-10-CM, was released in December 1997 and was available for comment for three months. The more than 1200 comments that were received were analyzed and categorized. Some comments were rejected, some were incorporated into ICD-10-CM, and some required further analysis for possible inclusion into ICD-10-CM. The preliminary analysis of ICD-10-CM was published in March 2003. These comments and preliminary analysis were posted on the NCHS Web site for further study. ICD-10-CM development has continued with further changes made in response to the open comment period as well as from physician specialty groups.

A pre-release draft version of ICD-10-CM was published on the NCHS Web site in June 2003 and included the Tabular List, Alphabetic Index, Neoplasm Table, External Cause of Injury Index, and Table of Drugs and Chemicals.

ICD-10-CM has the same type of hierarchy in its structure as ICD-9-CM. All codes have the same first three digits describing common traits, with each character beyond the first three providing more specificity. However, ICD-10-CM is alphanumeric with up to seven digits of specificity. ICD-10-CM also has the same organization and use of notes and instructions. When a note appears under a three-character code, it applies to all codes within that category, and notes under a specific code apply to the single code.

ICD-10-CM consists of the Alphabetical Index formatted by main terms listed in alphabetic order with indentations for any applicable qualifiers or descriptors. The Alphabetical Index is a list of terms with their corresponding codes. The Index is divided into two parts, the Index to Diseases and Injury and the Index to External Causes of Injury. Within the Index of Diseases and Injury there is the Neoplasm Table and a Table of Drugs and Chemicals.

The Tabular List is alphanumeric and groups diseases and injuries according to etiology (cause) or anatomical (body) site, which are listed in numeric order by diagnosis code. These groupings are organized into 21 chapters. The Tabular List groups injury and poisoning codes together (cause), whereas diseases that affect the respiratory system (anatomical site) are grouped together in another chapter.

The Neoplasm Table assists in the indexing and classification of neoplasms within ICD-10-CM. To properly code a neoplasm, it is necessary to determine from the record whether the neoplasm is benign, in situ, malignant, or of uncertain histologic behavior. If it is malignant, any secondary (metastatic) sites should also be determined.

The Table of Drugs and Chemicals in ICD-10-CM contains a classification of drugs and other chemical substances to assist in the reporting of poisoning, overdose states, and external causes of adverse effects.

The External Causes of Injury Index is a listing of external cause codes intended to provide data for injury research and evaluation of injury prevention strategies. These codes capture how the injury or health condition happened (cause), the intent (unintentional or accidental or intentional, such as suicide or assault), the place where the event occurred, and the activity of the patient at the time of the event.

The NCHS has continued to update ICD-10-CM (the latest update was published in 2009) along with the ICD-10-CM Official Guidelines for Coding and Reporting. The ICD-10-CM code set is located on the CMS Web site and can be downloaded at www.cms.hhs.gov/ICD10.

Replacing ICD-9-CM With ICD-10-CM

Discussions over replacing ICD-9-CM with ICD-10-CM began more than 10 years ago when the National Committee on Vital and Health Statistics (NCVHS) reported that ICD-9-CM was rapidly becoming outdated and recommended immediate US commitment to developing a migration to ICD-10 for morbidity and mortality coding. Since 1997, NCVHS has held more than eight days of hearings and received oral and written testimony from over 80 organizations representing the various stakeholders of the health care industry. NCVHS also commissioned the RAND Corporation to conduct an impact analysis study of moving to ICD-10-CM. The purpose of the analysis was to identify costs associated with the transition, information system changes, rate negotiation, reimbursement methodologies, training, forms changes, the impact of costs and benefits, and the potential return on the investment of implementation. NCVHS concluded, on the basis of the results of the RAND study and testimony, that ICD-10-CM should be adopted to replace ICD-9-CM and sent a letter to the secretary in 2003 recommending that HHS begin the regulatory process to adopt ICD-10-CM.

In addition, CMS recommended that steps be taken to improve the flexibility of ICD-9-CM or replace it with a more flexible option sometime after the year 2000. The final rule published on January 16, 2009, mandates conversion to ICD-10-CM on October 1, 2013.

The Benefits of Replacing ICD-9-CM With ICD-10-CM

ICD-10 contains an increased number of codes and categories that allow for more specific and accurate representation of current and future medical diagnoses and procedures. Because many other countries have already moved to ICD-10, we will be capturing morbidity data using the outdated classification system, ICD-9-CM.

Studies indicate that the United States needs to switch to ICD-10 in order to improve the quality of our nation's health care data and to maintain clinical data comparability. The longer we continue to use ICD-9-CM, the more difficult it becomes to compile and share accurate disease and mortality data at a time when such global data sharing is critical for public health. The better data provided by ICD-10 is expected to lead to improved patient safety, quality of care, and public health and bioterrorism monitoring.

There is a cost and a danger to using an outdated, "broken" coding system. Continuing to use ICD-9-CM will increasingly have an adverse impact on the value of health care data, including the accuracy of decisions based on faulty or imprecise data.

Take, for example, a patient who is seen by a physician and diagnosed with acute tonsillitis. This is the patient's second diagnosis of acute tonsillitis within the last six months.

In ICD-9-CM, acute tonsillitis is reported using ICD-9-CM code 463. There is no fourth or fifth digit in ICD-9-CM to identify the acute condition or the specific organism causing it.

In ICD-10-CM, the code set for tonsillitis is expanded to a fourth character extension to identify whether the acute condition is recurrent and the causative organism, if known.

Excerpt from ICD-10-CM (Acute tonsillitis)

J03   Acute tonsillitis

    J03.0   Streptococcal tonsillitis
        J03.00   Acute streptococcal tonsillitis, unspecified
        J03.01   Acute recurrent streptococcal tonsillitis

    J03.8   Acute tonsillitis due to other specified organisms
        J03.80   Acute tonsillitis due to other specified organisms
        J03.81   Acute recurrent tonsillitis due to other specified organisms

    J03.9   Acute tonsillitis, unspecified
        Follicular tonsillitis (acute)
        Gangrenous tonsillitis (acute)
        Infective tonsillitis (acute)
        Tonsillitis (acute) NOS
        Ulcerative tonsillitis (acute)
        J03.90   Acute tonsillitis, unspecified
        J03.91   Acute recurrent tonsillitis, unspecified

In ICD-10-CM, the patient encounter described above would be reported using code J03.91. More information is provided when the claim is submitted to the carrier to support medical necessity. More data is available to the insurance carrier in this example because the carrier knows this is a recurrent condition.

Rationale for Change

Very few unassigned codes remain in ICD-9-CM for accommodating new diagnoses. In addition to a lack of capacity for expansion, ICD-9-CM lacks accuracy in that many of the codes now in use do not accurately describe the diagnosis concepts they are assigned to represent. ICD-10-CM has the capability for expansion and more specificity in reporting diagnoses.

Although the United States has used ICD-10 coding to report mortality data since 1999, it still uses ICD-9 for reporting morbidities. This variation of data threatens our ability to track and respond to international threats to public health and bioterrorism. Rather than being a world leader in the collection of high-quality health data, the United States lags far behind.

At a time when the federal government is making significant progress toward improving our health information infrastructure, the critically needed upgrade to ICD-10-CM has been delayed with little acknowledgment of the serious consequences and no clear plan for fixing the problem. While the United States is working hard to adopt health information technology, it must also accommodate a robust 21st-century classification system.

Government and industry leaders cite health care initiatives that rely on data but are in fact compromised by the continued use of ICD-9-CM. These include quality measurement, pay-for-performance, medical error reduction, public health reporting, actuarial premium setting, cost analysis, and service reimbursement. Adoption of national electronic health records and interoperable information networks require improved classification systems for summarizing and reporting data.

Conversion to ICD-10-CM will not only produce better information and support further development of computer-assisted coding, it will serve as the necessary foundation for continued improvements and expansion of a 21st-century classification system, nationally and internationally.

Summary

For physician providers, ICD-10-CM will encompass more precise documentation of clinical care and will potentially ensure more accuracy when users determine medical necessity for the services provided. Our health care system faces quality concerns that are attributed to medical errors, poor documentation, lack of support of medical necessity, and fragmented care. This new system affords the opportunity for health care providers to code more accurately, which will contribute to health care quality improvement initiatives.

Resources

Graunt, J. *Natural and Political Observations Mentioned in a Following Index, and Made Upon the Bills of Mortality*. (Original work published 1662). Available online at www.edstephan.org/Graunt/0.html (accessed March 18, 2009).

American Health Information Management Association. *ICD-10-CM Field Testing Project*. Available online at www.ahima.org/icd10/documents/FinalStudy_000.pdf (accessed March 18, 2009).

Libicki M, Brahmakulam, I. RAND Science and Technology. *The Costs and Benefits of Moving to the ICD-10 Code Sets*. Available online at www.rand.org/pubs/technical_reports/2004/RAND_TR132.pdf (accessed March 18, 2009).

Nachimson Advisors. *The Impact of Implementing ICD-10 on Physician Practices and Clinical Laboratories: A Report to the ICD-10 Coalition*. Available online at http://nachimsonadvisors.com/Documents/ICD-10%20Impacts%20on%20Providers.pdf (accessed March 18, 2009).

Medicare Catastrophic Act of 1988. Available online at www.cbo.gov/ftpdocs/84xx/doc8430/88doc14.pdf (accessed March 18, 2009).

End-of-Chapter Questions

1   The clinical modification of ICD-9 (ICD-9-CM, Volumes 1 and 2), which is used today for reporting morbidities, was adopted in what year?

_____

2   The organization that conducted the impact analysis study for migration to ICD-10 is:

_____.

3   For physician providers, the realized benefits of ICD-10-CM include:

a.   _____

b.   _____

c.   _____

CHAPTER 3

Migration to ICD-10-CM

OBJECTIVES

- Review the potential costs for training in the use of the International Classification of Diseases, Tenth Revision, Clinical Modification (ICD-10-CM)
- Understand the need to identify business processes
- Understand the impact on loss of productivity during transition
- Understand the importance of reviewing health plan contracts
- Review the impact of increased time for documentation
- Review the impact on information technology systems
- Understand the potential impact on reimbursement
- Review the studies and reports on the impact of ICD-10-CM

Studies and Reports on ICD-10-CM

Many studies have been conducted as to whether ICD-10-CM will be of benefit to the health care industry. There are many challenges with implementing ICD-10-CM, including overall costs, system changes, business process changes, and training needs, and the list goes on. In 2003, the National Committee on Vital and Health Statistics requested that the RAND Corporation conduct a study of the costs and benefits of switching to ICD-10-CM. According to the RAND study, there are significant types of costs to providers, classified in these areas:

- Training physicians, coders, billers, and others
- Conducting process analysis
- Changing Superbills and encounter forms
- Documentation changes
- Loss of productivity
- Completing system changes
- Cash flow interruption.

Converting from ICD-9-CM to ICD-10-CM will impact not only individual providers but also hospitals, nursing homes, payers, software vendors, clearinghouses, and others, and much planning needs to be done prior to full implementation.

Training Costs

All involved organizations agree that in order to move effectively to ICD-10-CM, training is critical to the success of implementation. The cost of training physicians, coders, billers, and others will depend on the setting in which they work and their specific roles in their practices.

An American Health Information Management Association field study found that the time needed to retrain physicians, coders, billers, and others will be approximately four to eight hours. The ICD-10 final rule estimates that physicians and coders might need approximately 10 hours of training. This is the most significant coding change to occur in the past 30 years, and to assume that only 10 hours of training will be needed is inaccurate. In reality, according to the Nachimson report sponsored by the ICD-10 Coalition in October 2008, the learning curve for this transition might be quite steep for both clinical and administrative staff, especially in small to medium sized practices, which may not employ a certified professional coder. In-depth training will be required for clinical and administrative staff in regard to the following:

- Information technology
- Health insurance contracts
- Health plan policies
- Documentation
- Coding.

One should consider the time and costs of providing other continuing education to providers and staff. For an average practice, the cost for a one-day seminar on ICD-10-CM could be between $150 and $300 per attendee for a six-hour training session. However, a one-day training session may not provide adequate training for understanding ICD-10-CM fully. Other studies suggest training time may range from 16 to as many as 80 hours. There is considerable concern that coders will need to understand anatomy and physiology more extensively, which is not required for ICD-9-CM.

The United Kingdom, on the basis of its experience using ICD-10, recommended to the World Health Organization that, at a minimum, a coder should have 10 days of basic training involving a minimum of 70 hours.

The RAND study estimated that the cost of training for ICD-10-CM could be as high as $100 million nationally. However, taking into consideration that some staff will need more than four to eight hours of training, the costs could range from $50 million to $150 million.

The Nachimson study estimated that the typical small practice will spend a minimum of $2,405 for training clinical and administrative staff on ICD-10-CM, whereas a large practice might incur costs at well over $46,000.

One also must take into consideration that users may need time to understand guidelines and make themselves familiar with the codes. Physicians might rely on coders, or give them minimal training in order to understand the system, but regardless of the number of hours of training required, there will be costs involved to ensure the type of training necessary to use the new codes.

Clinical and administrative staff will initially need to understand the difference between ICD-9-CM and ICD-10-CM, along with the specific impact it will have on their practices. The learning curve is expected to be quite significant for both clinical and administrative staff, especially in small to medium sized practices that do not employ professional coders. Detailed training will be necessary for staff involved in the following:

- Coding of medical records
- Information technology

- Health plan relations
- Contracts
- Documentation of patient encounters.

Each practice will need to determine the number of people to send to training, along with what type of training methods they will employ. It is expected that many types of training will be available, such as courses, workshops, seminars, Web-based training, and audio conferences.

Overall, the amount of training required will depend on the role a staff person has in the practice. A coder might need 24 to 80 hours of coding-related training, whereas the physician might need only 10 to 12 hours of training. Nurses and nonclinical staff might need approximately 8 to 10 hours of training on the new code set.

The consequences for practices in which staff are not provided with training could be substantial. Without proper training, the productivity loss could be as high as six months to a year and could potentially result in a significant loss of revenue.

Another important consideration related to training is the timing of the training. Experience has shown that staff trained too early in the process will have forgotten much of the information by the final implementation date of October 1, 2013. If staff are trained too late, they may be overwhelmed by having the training and final steps of system implementation occurring at the same time. The exact timing of training will depend on the practice and the experience level of the staff. Approximately one year prior to the "go-live" date is considered to be an appropriate window for optimal staff training. This timing is to ensure everyone is trained. Some studies yielded conflicting recommendations for training. The American Hospital Association recommends starting three to six months before the go-live date. However, other organizations, such as the American Academy of Professional Coders, recommend that training begin as early as one year before the go-live date. The timeline in which the medical practice obtains training on ICD-10-CM code set will depend on the size of the organization and the amount of training required.

Cost of Process Analysis

Each practice should perform an analysis to determine how ICD-10-CM will impact its business processes. This step will be best accomplished by a manager or administrator of the practice who has obtained an initial understanding of ICD-10-CM. The analysis should identify what must be done to adapt to ICD-10-CM and should include a review of health plan contracts and a review of billing and coding procedures, such as the use of Superbills and encounter forms, patient procedures, and documentation.

The time it takes to complete this activity will depend on the size of the practice. A small practice might spend several weeks analyzing the process, whereas a large practice might spend several months.

Changes to Superbills and Encounter Forms

Even though many large practices are migrating to electronic medical records, many practices rely on Superbills and encounter forms to record procedures, services, and diagnoses. Typically, a practice will use the Superbill, which is a form listing their most common diagnosis codes, to speed up the code selection process at the time the patient is being seen.

As a result of the expansion of the number of diagnosis codes in ICD-10-CM, a paper Superbill or encounter form may become too lengthy to continue to serve its purpose of providing an efficient list of diagnosis codes. An electronic version might be necessary, which would negate the intent of having a simple paper process to assist with coding decisions at the time the patient is being seen. The paper Superbill or encounter form might become a thing of the past.

For example, in 2008, the American Academy of Family Practice conducted a study by converting the most common diagnoses used in a family practice environment to assess the impact of using a paper Superbill when the conversion to ICD-10-CM is complete. According to the new code sets, the Superbill or encounter form of an average family practice could expand to as many as nine pages. A nine-page form is unrealistic and would be too cumbersome and time consuming for the physician to use. An electronic Superbill might be an option for practices that do not plan to move to electronic medical records. Many electronic medical records incorporate the capture of the procedure and diagnosis codes to assist in the code selection process without the use of a paper Superbill.

If a practice decides to continue to use a paper Superbill, the cost of revising the Superbill, including staff time, outside vendor time, and expanded printing costs must be considered. With an electronic Superbill, the cost of the software, staff training, and additional time to use the system in the course of a patient's visit must be considered.

Increased Documentation

With the level of specificity in ICD-10-CM, additional detail might be necessary to support medical necessity when patient encounters are reported to health plans. This could lead to changes in the business process in a practice. Even though payment for professional services is driven by the procedure, the specificity of the diagnosis is important in supporting medical necessity and, therefore, is vital to payment of the health care claim.

Many instances of inaccurate coding arise from insufficient documentation in medical records, which may result in claim denials or payment reversals. When documentation in a medical record is not detailed enough, an unspecified diagnosis is reported. Many health plan policies require specific diagnoses to support medical necessity, so specificity is crucial. If a practice decides to continue to use unspecified codes with the ICD-10-CM conversion, this could result in rejected claims or claim suspension and health plans requesting more information.

Medical record documentation should support the diagnosis or procedure and ensure that services provided are consistent with patient symptoms and that they satisfy generally accepted medical standards. Physicians and other providers should ensure that the documentation for each patient encounter is adequate for coding and quality improvement purposes.

In preparation for ICD-10-CM, performing a documentation assessment of each physician and/or provider to ensure that the level of specificity is documented would be beneficial in assessing potential future reimbursement issues. This assessment could be accomplished either internally or externally by a qualified medical record reviewer. Costs to review and make changes to documentation could be substantial. The Nachimson report identified a potential 4% increase in provider work time for documentation changes.

Loss of Productivity

Loss of productivity must be another consideration both before and after implementation of ICD-10-CM. Coding itself is a process of translating words documented in the medical record into a numeric or alphanumeric code to support medical necessity for the service provided. These codes are sent either on a paper claim form or in an electronic claim to a health plan or third-party payer for payment and reimbursement.

ICD-10-CM has greater specificity, with up to seven character extensions, that will require a higher level of documentation. This may require providers to document additional information in support of the diagnosis reporting, as stated earlier. With the increased time it will take for documentation, there will be less time spent with patients.

One also must consider the loss of productivity when a staff member is out of the office for training. It could cost a practice, on average, $400 a day in lost productivity if a coder is out of the office. Staff members a practice needs to train include the following:

- Physicians
- Clinical staff
- Coders
- Billers
- Front office staff
- Managers and administrators
- Auditors/reviewers.

In many cases, both physicians and coders will need to communicate more closely, as additional information might be required to classify specific diagnoses. The RAND study estimated that the cost in lost productivity and time to resolve coding issues could range between $5 million and $25 million nationally for the first year and could decline to $16 million after 6 months. The amount of productivity lost in a practice depends on the level of understanding of ICD-10-CM and training obtained by the physician and staff.

The ICD-10 final rule addresses causes of productivity loss to include the following:

- Unfamiliarity with the index
- Use of different main terms and subordinate terms in ICD-10-CM versus ICD-9-CM
- Spending more time reviewing medical records
- Lack of familiarity with ICD-10-CM versus ICD-9-CM including guidelines, conventions, and the increased level of specificity.

It is safe to assume that these productivity losses could be as high as $30 million to $40 million for the first year after implementation, depending on the specialty and the complexity of coding associated with that specialty.

Even though it has been proven by many sources that greater specificity and detail in ICD-10-CM will, in the long term, reduce denials, submission of improper claims, and the number of requests by carriers for medical records, the initial transition might increase the number of rejections and denials. The increase in claim processing work by a practice may result in the need for staff to work overtime, raising costs as high at $20 million for the first year after implementation.

Information Technology System Changes

It is necessary to review the internal and external information technology system changes necessary for ICD-10-CM and to identify the systems that will be affected, including the following:

- Practice management systems
- Electronic medical record software
- Billing services
- Clearinghouses
- Other vendors.

Software modifications will be necessary to convert to the new code set. The crosswalk from ICD-9-CM to ICD-10-CM also must be considered. Even though the Centers for Medicare & Medicaid Services have developed a mapping system (see Chapter 9), each vendor will need to crosswalk and map the codes forward and backward. This means that mapping must be done forward (ICD-9-CM to ICD-10-CM) and backward (ICD-10-CM to ICD-9-CM) to process claims submitted prior to the final implementation date.

The amount of work that needs to be done depends on the size of the practice. For example, in a small practice, the practice management system and the electronic medical record software might be affected. But in a larger practice, other systems may be impacted. If the practice management system generates electronic transactions for eligibility and/or prior authorization, modifications to the system will be required.

If a practice uses a clearinghouse or billing service, it will be important for these entities to be prepared for ICD-10-CM to serve their clients. The development and testing of ICD-10-CM must be planned very carefully for information technology system vendors. All systems will need to be tested to ensure that the systems have been updated appropriately for the new code set. It is very likely that software changes will impact the business flow for a practice, which will necessitate training on system changes for all staff and clinicians. Hardware upgrades also must be taken into consideration. Using dual coding systems for a period of time after the transition might take up more hardware space than current systems can accommodate.

The Potential Impact on Reimbursement

To plan for the impact of conversion to ICD-10-CM on reimbursement, one must consider the number of claims a practice submits. For example, a surgical practice of three physicians that sees patients in the office three days per week, with two days in surgery, would submit approximately 87 claims per physician per week, making the estimated number of claims submitted 261 claims per week. If the number of claims submitted per week totals $145,000, loss of 10% to 25% of the practice's productivity would impact the bottom line and the overall financial health of the practice.

Many health care organizations in Canada reported a 10% decline in productivity in the years preceding and following implementation. The economic impact to all providers could be significant, with a risk of slower payments for three to six months. Three key areas that might be the cause of short-term productivity loss include the following:

- Queries from coders to clarify documentation in medical records
- Increased billing inquiries by payers
- Increased number of adjustments and pending or suspended claims.

Hiring additional trained staff to help with the backlog might be required because of the increased need to review charts and encounter forms to comply with documentation requirements.

With changes in the diagnostic coding system, many providers will be required to review and renegotiate their payer contracts, as many services are tied to reimbursement rates. Many of the policies are linked to diagnosis codes that support medical necessity for reimbursement. These policies will need extensive revision to map from the ICD-9-CM codes to the ICD-10-CM codes. Because of the number of third-party and commercial payer contracts, a significant amount of work and effort will be required prior to implementation so that reimbursement is not brought to a halt.

One may consider how the Centers for Medicare & Medicaid Services define National Coverage Determinations and Local Carrier Determinations. These policies will require review on the part of the medical practice to ensure that claims are submitted with the appropriate diagnosis codes.

Lessons Learned From Canada

Canada began implementation of the International Statistical Classification of Diseases and Related Health Problems, Tenth Revision, Canada (ICD-10-CA) and the Canadian Classification of Health Interventions in 2001. Canada chose to implement ICD-10-CA in phases, with five provinces and one territory as the first to migrate to ICD-10. More provinces converted between 2002 and 2006. To support the implementation, Canada created an education program of four modules, which included self-learning, a two-day workshop with a computer laboratory, on-line case studies for practice, and a one-day refresher course six months after the initial training.

Canada did not convert to ICD-10-CA without challenge. Two very common challenges the United States will face are the shortage of health professionals and resistance to change. Most coders in Canada had been in the profession for more than 20 years. This is typically true of the United States today. Canada could compare to the United States in that most coders, and physicians alike, know the most common diagnosis codes used in the practice by memory. One of the biggest challenges for the coders was forgetting the codes of the old code set that they had memorized. Coders must be retrained. Many coders in US physician practices sometimes fail to review the American Hospital Association's Coding Clinic reference and the Official ICD-9-CM Guidelines.

Another challenge Canada had is that during the transition, they switched to an electronic format of ICD-10-CA, and many people were not familiar with the electronic Alphabetic Index, so retraining on how to find the codes was required. Several provinces in Canada had difficulty filling jobs because of personnel shortages, and this created coding backlogs prior to and during implementation of the new classification.

Currently in the United States, there is a critical shortage of coders. According the Workforce Coding Professional Survey conducted by the American Health Information Management Association and the American Hospital Association, with support from the American Medical Association, over 76% of those responding to the survey reported difficulty in filling open positions with qualified skilled coders (www.ahima.org/emerging_issues/CodersWanted.pdf#page%3D2&search%3D%22Survey%22).

Because Canada implemented ICD-10-CA in the electronic environment, it impacted the difficulty of the transition. Productivity levels were also affected. On average, it took most health care environments a minimum of six months to get productivity to an acceptable level. Coders more comfortable with the electronic medium were able to make the transition quicker than those who were less comfortable with the medium. Even though Canada developed a group to help with the conversion, there was difficulty interpreting the data. Some of the major causative factors were the following:

- Coding rule changes
- New classification structure
- Conversion issues
- Coding and/or conversion errors.

However, Canada did identify some key benefits in migrating to ICD-10-CA. One key benefit was having one set of classification standards. Canada was using a variety of classifications, which presented obstacles in their national databases and in conducting interprovincial comparisons. Other benefits for Canada were having the same classification for inpatient and hospital-based ambulatory care, a more comprehensive scope, international comparability, and a more effective structure and presentation. One benefit of the ICD-10-CM structure is the number of available codes.

System Costs

It is understandable that the cost of converting information systems to ICD-10 will be enormous. The cost for implementation might be lower for medical practices, but every solo physician and group practice will be impacted. According to several studies, including the RAND Corporation Study, the study conducted by the Robert E. Nolan Company, and the Nachimson Advisor's White Paper, system upgrades overall for large practices, including clinical, scanning, billing, financial, and analysis software, could range from $500 million up to $1.6 billion nationally, with smaller or solo practices expected to spend $181 million overall. The cost would be a onetime system upgrade cost for the conversion.

A typical practice with three or more physicians might expect to spend between $2,000 and $8,000 for the conversion. A solo physician would likely spend between $1,000 and $4,000. Costs could be higher, depending on whether the systems vendor can upgrade the software and systems. If the practice management system is no longer being supported by the vendor or it could not be updated for technical reasons, the practice would need to purchase a new system. The purchase of a new system would likely be an unexpected expense.

Billing companies will likely either increase fees for their services or charge their clients a onetime upgrade fee. Depending on the size of the billing company, expenses for upgrading systems could range between $2,000 and $25,000 per organization.

Hospital implementation could cost an individual hospital from $100,000 up to $5 million, depending on the systems in place and the sizes of the organizations. These costs do not take into account other health care facilities, such as nursing homes and home health agencies. In all, the system-cost estimate for all ancillary providers (eg, durable medical equipment companies and laboratories) ranges between $200 million and $400 million nationally.

Software vendors will have the greatest challenge to convert their systems and products to meet the level of specificity in ICD-10. In addition, maps will need to be used for claims submitted prior to ICD-10 implementation. The vendor's work will require many resources and staff hours, which entails substantial costs that will likely be passed on to the client (ie, physician, hospital, or facility).

In addition, health plans, including Medicare and Medicaid, will need to upgrade their systems for ICD-10, and these costs have been estimated at between $100 million and $200 million as a whole and could escalate. It is likely that not every health plan will be ready on the go-live date. Nationally, on average, health plans could spend between $400 million and $800 million to implement ICD-10.

Pilot Testing of ICD-10-CM

The American Hospital Association in conjunction with the American Health Information Management Association conducted field testing of ICD-10-CM coding to determine whether this coding system would be applicable to actual medical record documentation and would be easy to learn by professional coders. Although a variety of health care providers was included in the pilot study, physician practices made up a small fraction of those participating, and hospital inpatient and outpatient providers made up the majority.

This project was conducted from June 30, 2003, to August 5, 2003. Participants were selected from all regions of the United States. The purpose of the field testing project was to assess the functionality and utility of applying ICD-10-CM to actual medical records in a variety of health care settings and to assess the level of education and training required by professional, credentialed coders to implement ICD-10-CM. There were 169 participants in the study, and each participant was required to complete a predetermined training program prior to participation with ongoing support from project coordinators. Each participant selected 50 records at random to code. The entire medical record was reviewed, and ICD-9-CM codes as well as ICD-10-CM codes were assigned to the patient encounter.

Resources used by the participants included the following:

- Training materials
- Coding guidelines
- Link to survey forms
- Ongoing communication between participants and project coordinators.

The process for the study included several items.

- The data collection period was from June 30, 2003, through August 5, 2003.
- Only discharged patient records were reviewed.
- Only completed medical records were used.
- Both ICD-9-CM and ICD-10-CM diagnosis codes were assigned for each record.
- The Official Guidelines for Coding and Reporting for ICD-9-CM and the draft guidelines for ICD-10-CM were used. The entire medical record was reviewed for each patient encounter.
- Participants assigned codes as completely and accurately as possible, according to existing medical record documentation.

Participants were instructed not to query the provider regarding unclear documentation. After completion of the project, each participant completed the following surveys.

- The demographic survey identified the participant's background, including credentials, certifications, experience level, and type of organization where employed.
- The record survey was completed once for each record coded. The participants identified the complexity and amount of time it took to code the medical record using ICD-9-CM versus ICD-10-CM.
- The follow-up survey was completed once at the conclusion of the project. The participants were asked their overall impression of ICD-10-CM, including the additional time it took to code the medical record, the level of complexity of ICD-10-CM, and their overall impression of the new code set.
- The supplemental survey was completed a few weeks after the conclusion of the project. It included the participants' overall impression of ICD-10-CM and their estimation of the level of coding training that would be needed once the conversion to ICD-10-CM was announced.

To validate the diagnostic information, every fifth record for half of the participants was recoded with additional data submitted, which comprised diagnoses documented in the medical record and the ICD-10-CM code assignment. The American Hospital Association and the American Health Information Management Association professional coding staff recoded validation forms in ICD-10-CM.

These data were submitted to Ohio State University for analysis and statistical tabulation. The University's health informatics and statistical staff cleaned the data and tabulated the results. The results were reported to the American Hospital Association and the American Health Information Management Association.

Records Coded

There were 6177 medical records coded, with only 6% from physician practices and 2.9% from clinics, community health centers, free-standing ambulatory surgery centers, and free-standing diagnostic facilities. Other records were coded from short-term, acute-care, inpatient settings (42.3%), short-term, acute-care, outpatient settings (38.8%), post-acute-care settings (7.9%), behavioral health facilities (1.6%), and other settings (0.6%). See Figure 3.1.

FIGURE 3.1 **Pilot Study Demographics by Facility or Type**	
Provider	**Percentage of Coded Records**
Short-term, acute-care, inpatient	42.3%
Short-term, acute-care, outpatient	38.8%
Post-acute-care settings	7.9%
Physician practices	6%
Clinics, community health centers, free-standing ambulatory surgery centers, freestanding diagnostic facilities	2.9%
Behavioral health facilities	1.6%
Other facilities	0.6%

The 6% of physician services coded resulted in 372 records, which is minimal in comparison to the 15,015 records coded for inpatient and outpatient short-term, acute-care hospital encounters. All participants had either a coding credential or a general health information management credential. The time the coders indicated they spent on coding medical records averaged from 25 to 40 hours a week in 25.5% of the group and one to five hours per week in 13.8% of the group. Participants included certified coders with the Certified Coding Associates (CCA), Certified Coding Specialist (CCS), and Certified Coding Specialist-Physician (CCS-P) credentials, comprising 14.2% of participants. The balance of participants in the study had Registered Health Information Administrator (RHIA) or Registered Health Information Technician (RHIT) credentials from the American Health Information Management Association.

Only 6% of the encounters coded were from medical practices. As a result, there was a limited amount of data for reporting professional services for physicians using ICD-10-CM.

The study indicates that ICD-10-CM should be implemented in three years or less. Most of the participants (60%) thought that 17 to 24 hours of training was all that was needed for implementation. However, only 6% of physician services were coded. Some participants thought that more in-depth training should be conducted so that fewer coding errors would occur. The participants agreed that ICD-10-CM is more detailed and would be a lot of coding information for the user to absorb. The majority of coders thought that three months prior to implementation would be a sufficient time frame for coding training, but that would not be enough time to assess the user's understanding of ICD-10-CM in most health care settings. Many large practices would need to begin the training process much earlier to ensure that everyone received adequate training and that there was sufficient time before implementation to conduct an assessment of users' understanding of the new code set.

Interestingly, most participants in the study thought that face-to-face training is more beneficial. Most professional coders agree that face-to-face training with an instructor who can answer questions and help clarify the gray areas is most effective, whereas with Internet-based training, audio seminars, or other types of training, the trainee might not receive this added benefit.

Some of the problems in coding ICD-10-CM in the study included conflicts in ICD-10-CM instructions and the use of nonspecific codes. Also problematic was that it took twice as long to assign an ICD-10-CM code as to assign an ICD-9-CM code. One of the problems identified was the minimal training the participants received prior to using the system and their unfamiliarity with the coding system. That assessment alone should validate the need for more extensive training on ICD-10-CM. Also problematic was the lack of user-friendly coding tools, which we have available with ICD-9-CM. Those tools will most likely be created either prior to or after implementation of ICD-10-CM. The amount of time to code an encounter should decrease as users become more familiar with the system. All coding problems in the study were reported to the National Center for Health Statistics for resolution.

One positive note is that even though documentation by physicians and nonphysician providers may not be as specific, it is easily corrected with training and ongoing reinforcement. Improved documentation would result in higher data quality and specificity, which would support medical necessity, reducing the number of claims reviewed.

In conclusion, the study was beneficial in identifying nonspecific codes, problems with unclear guidelines and instructions, and lack of tools needed to code effectively. The study also identified that training is required and productivity will be reduced during and after implementation until users are comfortable with the new coding system. The study overall determined how to assess (1) the functionality and utility of applying ICD-10-CM to actual medical records in a variety of health care settings and (2) the level of education and training required by professional, credentialed coders to implement ICD-10-CM.

Summary

The migration to ICD-10-CM will have a significant impact on clinical and business processes that will affect every organization in health care. This change will affect every aspect of the business, including quality measures, documentation, medical coverage, payment policies, productivity, and more. One-time costs will include upgrading information technology systems, changing Superbills and encounter forms, upgrading electronic health records, renegotiating commercial and managed care health plan contracts, and training.

Because payment to physicians is driven by insurance coverage and reimbursement policies, health plan coverage decisions will be based not only on procedures but also on medical necessity, interpreted from diagnosis codes. With the change to ICD-10-CM, payment delays could be expected with the code set change. Medical practices will need to stay updated on health plan policy changes to ensure reporting of correct ICD-10-CM codes.

Another area of concern is the loss of productivity while coders, clinicians, and other staff are undergoing training. The question of how offices will function when staff are in training must also be addressed. Coders will need more extensive training, whereas physician and nonphysician practitioners will need more specific training on the new classification system. Implementation costs will vary by practice size, number of training hours required, cost of training, and method of training obtained. Temporary staff might be necessary to keep the day-to-day operations running smoothly, which will be an additional cost.

In conclusion, the cost for implementation is a significant consideration, as are training, documentation, productivity issues, information technology system changes, and more. The stakeholders in medical practices large or small must complete a needs analysis to prepare for ICD-10-CM implementation.

Resources

Libicki M, Brahmakulam, I. RAND Science and Technology. *The Costs and Benefits of Moving to the ICD-10 Code Sets.* March 2003. Available online at www.rand.org/pubs/technical_reports/2004/RAND_TR132.pdf.

Nachimson Advisors, LLC. *The Impact of Implementing ICD-10 on Physician Practices and Clinical Laboratories: A Report to the ICD10 Coalition.* 2008. Available online at http://nachimsonadvisors.com/Documents/ICD-10%20 Impacts%20on%20Providers.pdf.

Robert E. Nolan Company. *Replacing ICD-9-CM with ICD-10-CM and ICD-10-PCS: Challenges, Estimated Costs and Potential Benefits.* 2003. Available online at www.renolan.com/knowledge/pastsurveys.htm.

American Health Information Management Association (AHIMA). *ICD-10 Field Testing Project Summary Report.* 2003. Available online at www.ahima. org/icd10/documents/FinalStudy_000.pdf.

End-of-Chapter Questions

1   According to the RAND study, there are three types of costs to providers. What are these potential costs?

    a. _____

    b. _____

    c. _____

2   Productivity might be impacted with ICD-10-CM implementation. Which three key areas might cause short-term productivity issues?

    a. _____

    b. _____

    c. _____

3   What two significant challenges might the United States have with ICD-10-CM implementation?

    a. _____

    b. _____

4   Why is diagnosis coding so important to the physician submitting claims

    for payment? _____

5   The American Health Information Management Association field testing study identified some problems with ICD-10-CM. What were they?

    a. _____

    b. _____

    c. _____

    e. _____

    f. _____

CHAPTER 4

Implementation of ICD-10-CM for Physicians and Staff

OBJECTIVES

- Review the steps for implementation of the International Classification of Diseases, Tenth Revision, Clinical Modification (ICD-10-CM)
- Understand the importance of documentation using ICD-10-CM
- Understand the steps in the training development plan
- Develop skills to identify budget needs, timelines, and the implementation process

Introduction

The ICD-10 final rule was published on January 16, 2009, and identified the timeline for implementing ICD-10-CM. The compliance date of October 1, 2013, is fast approaching. The time is now to begin the transition to ICD-10-CM for physicians and nonphysician providers. All practices, whether small or large, will be impacted by this change and need to begin early to ensure that when the go-live date arrives they are ready to begin claim submission with ICD-10-CM.

Obstacles to Overcome

One of the key obstacles to overcome is resistance to change. For many providers and coders, just finding the time to spend learning the new system will be difficult. The challenge of updating skills and learning a new system will be enough to drive some coders out of the profession. In addition to making the transition to ICD-10-CM, many practices are implementing electronic medical records (EMRs) or electronic health records, which adds to the complexity of change in a practice. On the positive side, the use of EMRs will add efficiency to a practice's documentation and billing processes because of greater specificity in the ICD-10-CM codes. The need to update skills is not limited to medical coders. Clinical staff also must be educated on ICD-10-CM, including the added level of specificity in the documentation.

In addition to training personnel, practices will need to update or change information systems, and the workflow and processes that many practices have been using for years may need to be changed or adjusted. There are many variables and issues to consider in moving to ICD-10-CM. This will be one of the largest changes to impact the health care industry in 20 years. Waiting until the last minute will impact a practice's livelihood and financial stability. The time to begin preparing for this massive undertaking is today.

It is important to begin the implementation process step by step. One cannot focus on all elements that need to be addressed at one time. Practices should begin by systematically focusing on one step at a time and creating a timeline to phase in ICD-10-CM. The amount of work necessary to implement ICD-10-CM and the resources required will depend on the size of the practice. A large practice may need to recruit key persons from many different departments and areas of the practice to assist with the transition, whereas a small practice might incorporate only one or two persons to assist in the transition. The process of conversion to ICD-10-CM may be similar to those used to implement similar projects, such as the electronic transactions required under the Health Insurance Portability and Accountability Act.

Key Steps in ICD-10-CM Implementation

Implementation of ICD-10-CM will take a systematic approach. Implementation not only involves learning the new code set, but many other areas prior to learning the codes. Planning and implementation of ICD-10-CM will need to include communication and significant collaboration in information technology, finance, clinical areas, payers, and outcomes. The following key steps should be taken in implementing ICD-10-CM.

1   Organize a project team and resources for project completion.

2   Conduct a preliminary impact analysis.

3   Create an implementation timeline.

4   Develop an ICD-10-CM implementation budget.

5   Analyze documentation needs.

6   Develop a communication plan.

7   Develop a training plan.

8   Complete information systems design and development.

9   Conduct a business process analysis.

10   Conduct a needs assessment.

11   Complete deployment of the system changes.

Step 1: Organize a Project Team and Resources for Project Completion

The first step is to create a project team within the practice to begin the planning process. The project team can be a committee or a single person, depending on the size of the practice. If the practice chooses to establish a committee, the committee should include at least one physician, the administrator or manager, coders, billers, and other key staff members. If the practice is small, it might involve only the manager, physician, and coder or a single person, such as the office manager.

It is important to have the physicians involved so they understand the importance of preparation as migration to ICD-10-CM occurs. A practice also needs physician support for successful implementation.

The project team should meet initially to begin to identify the elements for implementation. The team will need to establish an outline for ICD-10-CM implementation items to be addressed. A large practice will have many items to address, whereas a small or solo practice may have fewer issues to tackle. A small practice might benefit from hiring a consultant to either participate in the project or coordinate the overall transition plan. In a large practice, leadership staff should be involved in the development of the transition plan.

The project team should begin with key areas of focus in:

- preparing a project summary that includes an overview description of the project and anticipated work to be done;
- identifying leadership staff to oversee the project;
- establishing leadership's role in completing the project;
- establishing a line of communication to report the process with implementation;
- conducting a preliminary impact analysis;
- assessing current areas for documentation improvement;
- developing an implementation timeline;
- reviewing budget planning;
- identifying the systems that will be affected (eg, practice management system or EMR);
- training practitioners, coders, billing staff, and other identified staff;
- identifying resources to map from ICD-9-CM to ICD-10-CM specific to the practice specialty;
- working with information systems or vendors on issues related to coding specifications (ie, six-digit and seven-digit character extensions, alphanumeric format);
- orienting the physicians and clinical staff on how the system can be used by the practice;
- reviewing the impact on and expectations for documentation;
- reviewing and updating coding support tools such as Superbills;
- discussing with vendors when to expect software updates and what the estimated costs will be;
- identifying the overall impact on ICD-10-CM related to office work processes;
- assessing coding personnel's skills to identify knowledge gaps in the areas of medical terminology, anatomy and physiology, pathophysiology, and pharmacology to ensure that expanded clinical knowledge meets ICD-10-CM requirements;
- identifying weaknesses for which additional education would be beneficial;
- identifying communication methods for staff not involved in the project team and developing a communication plan to keep others informed of the ongoing work; and
- reviewing current health plan policies.

Once the project team is set, it is time to get to work. The first step is preparing a project summary, including an overview description of the regulation, changes to the code set, and anticipated internal and external work processes. For larger practices this could mean reading the ICD-10 final rule; for smaller practices this could mean reading materials prepared by a professional society. The project summary, along with an outline of project steps, will serve as the roadmap for completing the implementation. Every practice should begin this process immediately. Preparing for this change will take a great deal of time and effort.

The project team will be instrumental in the success of implementing ICD-10-CM and should be proactive in its preparation. All staff members should be involved in some way in the transition to ICD-10-CM. It is important to understand that the transition effort will not succeed without input and cooperation from all members of the practice. Personnel involved in the transition process should begin planning early to avert problems in the process.

One of the main concerns with this implementation is the delay of claim submission resulting from the learning process with ICD-10-CM. It is a fact that people's productivity decreases short term when they are in training or learning a new skill. These slowdowns result in loss of productivity, including charge capture and reimbursement, and can affect the financial health of a practice. The project team should anticipate a decrease in productivity by measuring and analyzing the impact of the transition prior to beginning the training process.

Step 2: Conduct a Preliminary Impact Analysis

It is important to determine how each practice will be impacted by ICD-10-CM by identifying which departments or areas will be affected and how they will be affected. The areas that will be impacted most significantly will be the information systems, practice management system, and/or EMR system. The project team should analyze how the practice is using these systems and determine whether these systems can be upgraded to ICD-10-CM. Calling system vendors may be necessary, and this may help determine whether the practice needs to upgrade hardware and software to accommodate ICD-10-CM.

How will patient care be impacted? Will it take more time for a physician to document more specificity to support medical necessity so claims are paid appropriately? Will each patient encounter take more time because of the expansion of the specificity of ICD-10-CM? This might impact the number of patients a physician can see each day. Consider the current information systems used in the practice. A small practice might have a practice management system and coding tools, such as encoders or code look-up programs. A large practice might have an EMR system integrated into the practice management system, a charge master, and other financial programs tied into the coding.

Another element to analyze is the coding skill set of the physicians, clinical staff, and coding and billing staff. Who assigns the ICD-9-CM codes to the patient encounter? If the physician is assigning the diagnosis code, office work flow may change with ICD-10-CM. If the practice is using EMRs, the impact might not be as significant, but if the practice is using a Superbill, the expansion of the diagnosis codes may create a problem. The project team should review how the staff is currently trained on coding and kept updated on health plan policies. How will this change impact time and resources required for the transition?

IMPLEMENTATION TIP

Communication with all physicians and staff will help to ensure a smooth transition. It is necessary to keep all staff informed of the ongoing work and transition dates.

Practices should review current health plan policies. Local and national coverage policies might change with ICD-10-CM. That might impact treatment protocols. Most health plan policies do include diagnoses that support medical necessity for the services provided.

If a practice is using a Superbill to record procedures and diagnoses, the Superbill should be reviewed and compared to the ICD-10-CM codes. Will the practice continue using the Superbill, or will the expansion of codes make the Superbill too cumbersome to use? The one-page Superbill will become a thing of the past because most ICD-10-CM code categories contain more specificity and 10 times as many diagnosis codes. A seven- or eight-page Superbill may be impractical. A practice might investigate other options, such as an electronic version of a Superbill. It is most certain that software vendors are analyzing this option for practices that choose not to migrate to the EMR soon. An electronic Superbill might also benefit practices that are using the EMR.

It will be evident, on the basis of the preliminary impact analysis, that every aspect of a practice will be affected, including documentation, information technology systems, coding, record keeping processes, fee schedules, medical review edits by health plans, and quality measurements that are used to assess performance.

Step 3: Create an Implementation Timeline

Implementation of ICD-10-CM will take a minimum of four years. Transition to ICD-10-CM will be a major disruption to the day-to-day operations of a practice for both administrative and clinical staff. Having an implementation timeline in place with key elements that need to be accomplished with milestones is imperative for a smooth transition. The timeline should encompass the whole transition and be further divided into each year. The timeline and milestones will be easier to track if broken down by year.

Each practice's timeline might look different depending on the size and scope of the practice's impact analysis. From the preliminary impact analysis, it should be evident to the practice, regardless of size, which elements will be impacted. The practice timeline should have a four-year budget, with implementation spread over that period, to lessen the financial impact of the transition.

Most practices rely more heavily on vendors than large hospital systems do. Vendors provide hardware and software for the practice management system, EMR, and other software programs used. A practice must begin work early with the vendors to determine:

- what implementation plans vendors have in place for the conversion;
- what products and services will be available;
- how long software development will take;
- when vendors will be ready to begin testing and implementing their products and services in the practice;
- when vendors will schedule installation; and
- what guidance and assistance vendors will provide during the rollout.

Software vendors may have thousands of customers to serve, and the sooner the practice makes contact and gets on a vendor's schedule, the easier the transition will be.

It is a good idea to divide the timeline into three- or four-year increments. If a practice begins the implementation process in 2009, tasks can be spread out so as not to substantially impact patient care.

Review Figures 4.1 to 4.4, which are examples of potential timelines for a medical practice for implementation of ICD-10-CM in four years.

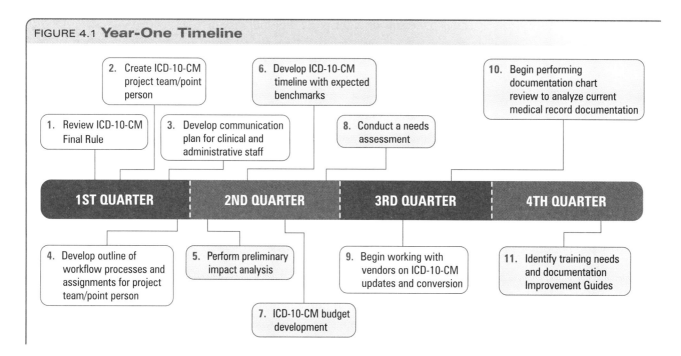

FIGURE 4.1 **Year-One Timeline**

2. Create ICD-10-CM project team/point person

6. Develop ICD-10-CM timeline with expected benchmarks

10. Begin performing documentation chart review to analyze current medical record documentation

1. Review ICD-10-CM Final Rule

3. Develop communication plan for clinical and administrative staff

8. Conduct a needs assessment

1ST QUARTER   **2ND QUARTER**   **3RD QUARTER**   **4TH QUARTER**

4. Develop outline of workflow processes and assignments for project team/point person

5. Perform preliminary impact analysis

9. Begin working with vendors on ICD-10-CM updates and conversion

11. Identify training needs and documentation Improvement Guides

7. ICD-10-CM budget development

In Figure 4.1, the timeline for year one is the preliminary planning phase. The activities in the planning phase include conducting a preliminary practice analysis, developing the timeline, developing the budget, performing a needs assessment, consulting with vendors, performing chart reviews to assess the current status of documentation, identifying training needs for documentation improvement, and formulating a plan to communicate the project status to the staff.

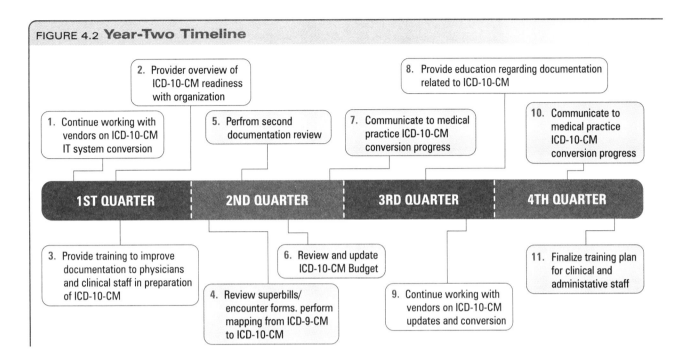

FIGURE 4.2 **Year-Two Timeline**

Year two (Figure 4.2) includes continuous communication of ICD-10-CM implementation development to staff, along with continued communication with vendors. Documentation reviews and education targeted for improvements can be completed with providers. The budget should be reviewed and updated with any additional costs expected. The training plan for staff should also be finalized.

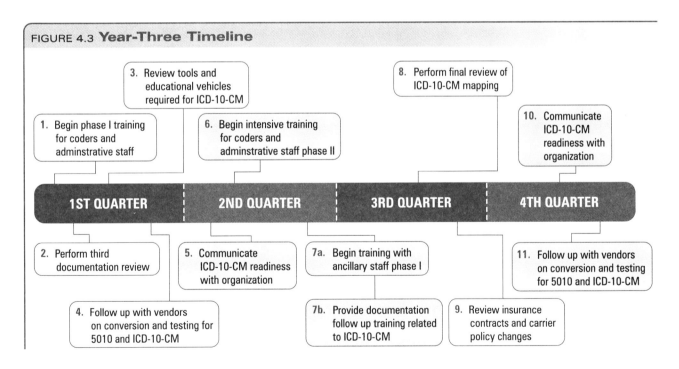

FIGURE 4.3 **Year-Three Timeline**

In year 3 (Figure 4.3), the timeline should include phase I training for all staff, a third documentation review, continued follow-up with vendors, a review of Superbills and encounter forms with mapping to ICD-10-CM, a review of educational resources the practice will need with ICD-10-CM, and a review of health plan contracts and any policy changes.

Year 4 (Figure 4.4) will be the most intensive phase of preparing for ICD-10-CM implementation. Activities will include testing the ICD-10-CM conversion with vendors or information technology staff, phase II training for staff, and continued communication with the staff. A performance outcomes measurement to assess the staff's understanding of ICD-10-CM should occur in this phase, in addition to any follow-up or retraining prior to implementation.

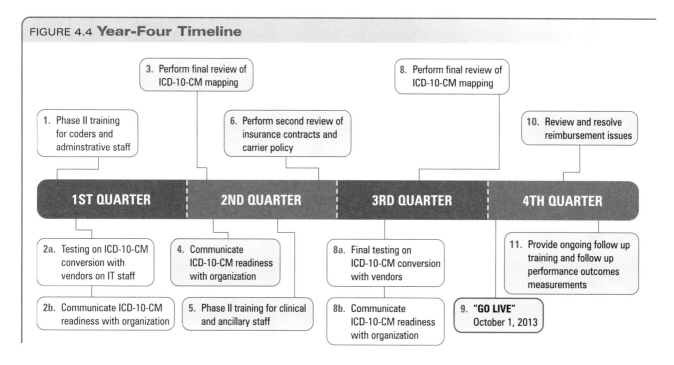

FIGURE 4.4 **Year-Four Timeline**

Each timeline will look different, on the basis of the size of the practice and the timeline the practice develops.

Step 4: Develop an ICD-10-CM Implementation Budget

Budget planning is an important step in the implementation process. This task might take some research and discussion with various vendors. In this early stage of implementation, the budget is a projection or estimate of potential costs. It can be as simple as creating a spreadsheet with items and services necessary for implementation. The project may be completed in phases, so a two-year budget plan would be less painful to the practice than a last-minute conversion.

The cost for implementation will depend on the size of the practice. The largest expenditure is expected to include the practice management system and EMR. The cost to upgrade systems could be minimal, or it could amount to thousands of dollars, depending on the systems in use, the size of the practice, and current contracts with vendors. Budgeting for ICD-10-CM should be spread out at a minimum over a three-year period, because implementation will be costly for any size practice. Careful analysis of costs will be critical in developing an ICD-10-CM implementation budget.

The following items should be considered in budget development:

- Software and licensing costs
- Hardware procurement
- Development costs
- Implementation deployment costs
- Possible EMR upgrade costs
- Staff training costs
- Overtime costs due to training other staff
- Cost to update Superbill/encounter forms
- Work flow process changes costs
- Testing costs.

It is important in developing a budget for ICD-10-CM implementation to communicate the budget plan with the appropriate key people within the practice. This is imperative for success of the implementation process.

Many organizations have estimated costs for ICD-10-CM implementation for small to large practices. A typical small practice with three to five physicians could experience a total expenditure of approximately $40,000 or more, according to the RAND Corporation study, the Nolan study, and the Hay Group study. Cost varies from study to study, but it is evident that the transition to ICD-10-CM will be costly for every practice in the country.

On average, a practice should plan to spend between $4,000 and $10,000 for system upgrades, depending on the systems used in the practice. A very large practice could spend over $100,000 for information technology system costs alone. Practices should contact their practice management software vendors to obtain the estimated cost immediately when preparing the budget.

Practices using an EMR should contact their software vendors to find out what software update costs will be. Upgrades to other systems that might affect coding should also be considered.

Figure 4.5 is a sample budget for a small surgical practice of three physicians.

FIGURE 4.5 Sample Budget for a Small Surgical Practice

INFORMATION SYSTEMS		ESTIMATED	ACTUAL
Practice management system		$4,000.00	
Electronic medical record		$3,000.00	
Coding software		$1,000.00	
Totals		**$8,000.00**	**$0.00**

AUDITING/REVIEW/MAPPING	ESTIMATED TIME	ESTIMATED	ACTUAL
General consulting/audit year 1		$6,000.00	
General consulting/audit year 2		$6,000.00	
General consulting/training		$3,000.00	
Review of system process	15 hours	$3,000.00	
Mapping to ICD-10-CM	30 hours	$6,000.00	
Totals		**$24,000.00**	**$0.00**

TRAINING		ESTIMATED TIME	ESTIMATED	ACTUAL
Physicians	3	20 hrs @ $1,000 per	$3,000.00	
Coders	1	60 hrs @ $3,000 per	$3,000.00	
Managers	1	20 hrs @ $1,000 per	$1,000.00	
Nurses	3	10 hrs @ $500 per	$1,500.00	
Ancillary staff	1	10 hrs @ $500 per	$500.00	
Totals			**$9,000.00**	**$0.00**

OVERTIME	ESTIMATED TIME	ESTIMATED	ACTUAL
Coders	60 hrs pre- and postimplementation	$2,500.00	
Ancillary staff	10 hrs pre- and postimplementation	$500.00	
Totals		**$3,000.00**	**$0.00**

TOTALS		ESTIMATED	ACTUAL
Information systems		$8,000.00	
Consulting/auditing/mapping		$24,000.00	
Training		$9,000.00	
Overtime		$3,000.00	
Total estimated expenses		**$44,000.00**	**$0.00**

Figure 4.6 is an example of a typical medium practice with 10 physicians.

FIGURE 4.6 ICD-10-CM Implementation Budget Worksheet, Two-Year Budget

INFORMATION SYSTEMS		ESTIMATED	ACTUAL
Practice management system		$8,000.00	
Electronic medical record		$6,000.00	
Coding software		$2,000.00	
Totals		**$16,000.00**	**$0.00**

AUDITING/REVIEW /MAPPING	ESTIMATED TIME	ESTIMATED	ACTUAL
General consulting/audit year 1		$10,000.00	
General consulting/audit year 2		$10,000.00	
General consulting/training		$6,000.00	
Review of system process	15 hours	$4,000.00	
Mapping to ICD-10-CM	30 hours	$6,000.00	
Totals		**$36,000.00**	**$0.00**

TRAINING		ESTIMATED TIME	ESTIMATED	ACTUAL
Physicians	10	20 hrs @ $1,000 per	$10,000.00	
Coders	4	60 hrs @ $3,000 per	$12,000.00	
Managers	1	20 hrs @ $1,000 per	$1,000.00	
Nurses	8	10 hrs @ $500 per	$4,000.00	
Ancillary staff	3	10 hrs @ $500 per	$1,500.00	
Totals			**$28,500.00**	**$0.00**

OVERTIME	ESTIMATED TIME	ESTIMATED	ACTUAL
Coders	60 hrs pre- and postimplementation	$9,500.00	
Ancillary staff	10 hrs pre- and postimplementation	$3,000.00	
Totals		**$12,500.00**	**$0.00**

TRAINING		ESTIMATED	ACTUAL
Information systems		$16,000.00	
Consulting/auditing/mapping		$36,000.00	
Training		$28,500.00	
Overtime		$12,500.00	
Total estimated expenses		**$93,000.00**	**$0.00**

Once a good assessment of potential costs for system changes is determined, a practice should look at the costs for mapping, consultants, and training. It is recommended that practices include consulting services in the budget costs. Consulting services may range from $150 to $200 an hour on average for a consultant to work with the practice for a timely and seamless transition to ICD-10-CM.

Mapping the ICD-9-CM codes to ICD-10-CM codes will be a time-consuming task. How a practice uses ICD-9-CM currently must be considered. If the practice is using a Superbill or encounter form to capture ICD-9-CM codes during the patient encounter, the Superbill will need to be mapped to ICD-10-CM.

The Superbill will need to be reviewed along with utilization of ICD-9-CM codes from the practice management system. Compiling a report from the practice management system will give the practice an understanding of the most frequently used ICD-9-CM codes. Typically, a Superbill that includes ICD-9-CM codes is not always up-to-date and/or the physicians do not use all the codes on the form. Reviewing what is currently on the Superbill will help update the current form and streamline its use for ICD-10-CM. Budget costs for Superbill review, utilization review, and mapping should be included when the ICD-10-CM budget is created. The review could take between 20 and 30 hours to complete. If a practice is small, it might benefit from having an outside source, such as a consultant or vendor, to develop the code mapping.

Small practices with limited resources may want to use a consultant to complete the mapping work, which will take many hours. If the practice is medium to large in size, the practice might have staff to perform the mapping from ICD-9-CM to ICD-10-CM. Even though the Centers for Medicare & Medicaid Services (CMS) have developed a mapping mechanism called General Equivalence Mappings, or GEMs, it will still take time to complete this task.

Training will be a large expenditure and should be analyzed carefully. Development of the training plan might take 10 to 15 hours to complete. There are many issues to consider in developing a training plan. Who will require training? First and foremost, the physicians, nurse practitioners, and physician assistants will need to be trained as well as nurses, medical assistants, and other clinical staff. Of course the coders, billers, and managers will need training as well as the front office and ancillary staff. A practice might even want to include the costs for additional chart audits to make sure the documentation will support diagnosis coding for ICD-10-CM, once practitioners receive the appropriate education and training.

Other questions to consider include the following. How much training is needed, and what are the costs? How many days of training will be required? What about lost revenue if the physicians and nonphysician practitioners need to be out of the office for training? How will productivity be affected? These are all valid concerns and need to be part of the budget planning process. When training costs are considered, a practice should determine how much training each department or staff person needs.

Physicians, nonphysician practitioners, coders, and billing staff might need more extensive training than ancillary staff (eg, nurses, front office staff). Training time and costs depend on the role of the staff person in the practice.

Everyone in the practice will need some form of training. Consider a medium-sized surgical practice with 10 physicians, two nurses, two coders/billers, one manager or administrator, and three office staff (receptionist, scheduler, and authorization specialist). The physicians will need approximately 16 to 20 hours of training. Nurses will probably need an introduction to ICD-10-CM, and 6 to 10 hours of training for this should be sufficient. The coders will need between 40 and 60 hours of training, and the ancillary staff will need 6 to 10 hours of training. Keep in mind that the number of hours of training depends on individuals' understanding of anatomy and medical terminology and their current understanding of ICD-9-CM. A person experienced in ICD-9-CM coding who has a good understanding of anatomy and medical terminology in the specialty may take less time to train than a person with limited knowledge.

Overtime is another expenditure to consider. Physicians and managers are most likely compensated on the basis of revenue or salary, so overtime will not be a consideration for them. However, coders and ancillary staff are typically paid an hourly rate. It is recommended to budget a minimum of 15 to 20 hours preimplementation and 20 to 40 hours postimplementation for overtime. After implementation, the amount of work will increase due to system problems, health plan claim denials, and other items that will need to be addressed, along with the daily business that occurs in the typical practice.

When the budget is created, estimations should be made at the higher costs, because there will always be unexpected costs that will occur with implementation. Once a practice has a good idea of estimated costs, it is time for the project team to develop a timeline for ICD-10-CM implementation. One idea is to use a spreadsheet to map a three-year plan for completing this monumental project.

Think about how diagnosis codes are used in the practice. Typically, a practice uses diagnosis codes in its practice management system, EMR, Superbills, and other documents and systems. There will be costs to upgrade or replace the system software along with changes to the Superbill and work flow processes. New hardware might be needed to accommodate the upgrade or replacement of the software because of the size of ICD-10-CM. Also consider that once the conversion takes place, ICD-9-CM codes will need to be maintained in the system(s) for outstanding claims submitted prior to the implementation date.

The practice will also need to consider areas for documentation improvement and the cost to review documentation to make sure the specificity will be achieved for ICD-10-CM. In a practice of three to five physicians, the cost would average $6,000 for one audit, with the probability of more than one audit in the two-year implementation period. Costs could escalate if ongoing education and training are needed to support compliance with diagnosis documentation in medical records.

Once the preliminary impact analysis and budget are finalized, the next step is to review the current documentation. It is beneficial to first analyze current documentation to determine whether the documentation will support ICD-10-CM. This will help the practice understand what changes must be made prior to implementation. With the increase in number of codes and specificity, it might be necessary for more detailed documentation in patient medical records to support treatment plans.

IMPLEMENTATION TIP

A good rule of thumb is to create a budget for the transition and break it down per year, so expenditures can be spread over at least a three-year period.

Step 5: Analyze Documentation Needs

Each practice should take an in-depth look at the current level of documentation in its medical records, then review areas for improvement in specificity of the documentation and analyze how to begin the process of improvement. The diagnosis codes used most commonly and the frequency of their use, based on the specialty of the practice, should be reviewed. Most practice management billing software is capable of producing a frequency report of diagnosis codes. This is useful for reviewing diagnosis code utilization in the practice.

In the past, practitioners used documentation in medical records to document the patient's problems and conditions. However, in recent years, medical records have become a tool to document medical histories as well as to provide a method by which health statistics are tracked. Medical records also act as legal documents, justify to health plans the charges billed on the basis of the medical care provided, and provide information for assessing quality of care.

Medical records are currently kept in either paper or electronic format. Some examples of types of services found in the medical record are the following:
- Outpatient office visits
- Consultations
- Medications and prescriptions
- Immunization records
- Laboratory tests and results
- Radiographs, imaging, and diagnostic studies
- Surgical services and operative reports
- Hospital records
- Pathology services.

Organization and maintenance of medical records is an important factor in providing quality care. A well-organized and well-maintained medical record will provide a more user-friendly source of information for internal staff, physicians, auditors, and insurance carriers.

Now is the time to perform a baseline ICD-10-CM readiness audit. Why is performing an audit so important? In order to move readiness forward, it is important to identify current areas for improvement in documentation when reporting diagnoses in medical records.

Many practices have staff who conduct audits or routinely have a consultant audit medical records for appropriate documentation and coding. This is a very important element of compliance, and many practices have undergone this process from a comprehensive coding perspective. However, what actually needs to be done is to review the patient chart to make sure the physician or nonphysician practitioner is documenting a complete diagnosis.

For example, if a patient presents with ear pain, and the physician performs and documents an assessment including a history pertinent to the reason for the visit, an examination, and medical determination based on the patient's history and examination, the diagnosis is likely to be documented as *acute otitis media* without further elaboration. The diagnosis code reported in ICD-9-CM would be unspecified (381.00, unspecified acute nonsuppurative otitis media).

However, in ICD-10-CM, the diagnosis of acute otitis media (H65.1-other acute nonsuppurative otitis media) cannot be coded without additional information such as what ear is affected and identification of whether the problem is initial or recurrent. More information must be documented in the medical record to support selection of an ICD-10-CM code. The documentation should look more like this: "Patient has an acute onset of otitis media of the right ear, which is recurrent." This information can be coded with ICD-10-CM using H65.114 (Acute and subacute otitis media recurrent, right ear).

Using ICD-10-CM coding is more specific because to code correctly, more information is needed, such as whether the condition is acute or subacute and which ear is affected.

The medical record is the primary means of communication between health care providers. Because the medical record is the main source of health information, it is imperative to maintain accurate, comprehensive, and appropriately coded data. Also, a properly documented medical record is essential to good quality patient care. With clinical coding, a number is assigned to diagnoses for retrieval, research, and reimbursement. Within the coding process, the coder will:

- review the medical record;
- select the items to code;
- assign the appropriate code(s);
- sequence the code(s) according to coding guidelines;
- abstract and enter the data into a database; and
- store and retrieve the coded data in a database.

Accurate diagnosis coding cannot be achieved without clear and complete documentation. Documentation will be critical with the adoption of ICD-10-CM in the United States. The new classification system contains a significant increase in the number of codes, compared with ICD-9-CM, and some sections have been added or revised. Even though the two diagnosis coding systems are parallel, documentation may require more attention, because the documentation must contain more detail for assignment of the appropriate codes.

For example, a patient presented to his family practitioner with asthma that has acutely exacerbated. The physician documented acute asthma in the medical record and ordered a nebulizer treatment. In ICD-9-CM, the code could be easily identified as 493.92: Asthma, unspecified, with (acute) exacerbation.

Using ICD-10-CM, selecting an appropriate diagnosis with the documentation is more difficult because more information is required. Compare the difference between ICD-9-CM and ICD-10-CM in Figure 4.7. In order to code the same diagnosis in ICD-10-CM, further documentation is required to indicate whether the asthma is:

- mild, intermittent with acute exacerbation;
- moderate, persistent, with acute exacerbation; or
- severe, persistent, with acute exacerbation.

FIGURE 4.7 ICD-9-CM and ICD-10-CM Diagnoses for Asthma With an Acute Exacerbation (GEMs File)

ICD-9-CM Code(s)		ICD-10-CM Code(s)	
493.02	Asthma, unspecified, with (acute) exacerbation	J45.21	Asthma, mild, intermittent w/acute exacerbation
		J45.41	Asthma, moderate, persistent, with (acute) exacerbation
		J45.51	Asthma, severe, persistent, with (acute) exacerbation

Code selection is based on more detailed information. With the information documented in the example, code selection would be more difficult. ICD-10-CM will provide a clearer clinical picture, which will support medical necessity more definitively.

Review the previous example again, now that documentation improvements efforts have been completed: A patient presented to his family practitioner with severe persistent asthma acutely exacerbated, and the physician ordered a nebulizer treatment. Now the patient encounter can be coded with ICD-10-CM. The encounter is coded as J45.51: Asthma, severe, persistent, with (acute) exacerbation.

Review the following example along with Figure 4.8: A patient presented with varicose veins of the right and left legs with calf ulceration limited to skin breakdown on the right and pain on the left.

In this example, it is possible to code using both ICD-9-CM and ICD-10-CM because the documentation in the medical record is sufficient. Review the code comparison in Figure 4.8.

FIGURE 4.8 ICD-9-CM and ICD-10-CM Diagnoses for Varicose Veins

ICD-9-CM Code(s)		ICD-10-CM Code(s)	
454.0	Varicose veins of lower extremities with ulcer	I83.012	Varicose veins of right lower extremity with ulcer of calf
454.8	Varicose veins with other complications	I83.812	Varicose veins of left lower extremities with pain
707.12	Ulcer of calf	L97.211	Non-pressure chronic ulcer of right calf limited to breakdown of skin

Notice in Figure 4.8 that the three codes that map to ICD-9-CM in ICD-10-CM have more specificity in reporting the documented diagnosis. Using ICD-9-CM, diagnosis code 454.0 is used to report the varicose veins of both lower extremities along with the secondary diagnosis of 702.12 for the calf ulceration. ICD-10-CM uses two codes, I83.012 and I83.812, to report the varicose veins of the left and right lower extremities, and code L97.211 is reported as a secondary diagnosis to identify the specific site and severity of the ulcer.

FIGURE 4.9 **Code Comparison for Varicose Veins**

ICD-9-CM Code(s)	ICD-10-CM Code(s)
• Pain included in the "other" complication group • Combination codes for complications but not to the location • Unable to identify the severity of the ulcer	• Expansion of combination codes for varicose veins and associated complications with the addition of a specific subclassification for pain • Codes specify laterality • Codes specify the site of the ulcer • Codes specify the severity of the ulcer

Because all health care providers will be required to document descriptive detail in order to facilitate correct coding, it is recommended that each practice consider evaluating strengths and weaknesses in its current documentation and make the necessary changes to ensure a smooth transition to ICD-10.

ICD-10-CM is more comprehensive than ICD-9-CM and equates more closely with the vocabulary and practice of current medicine. This enables more detailed and accurate classification of diseases, which leads to more efficient and effective data retrieval.

Improvements in the ICD-10-CM content include more detailed information on ambulatory and other subacute and nonacute care encounters; expanded injury codes; combination diagnosis/symptom codes, which will reduce the number of codes needed to fully describe a condition; laterality; and a more consistent method of coding postprocedural conditions. In addition, ICD-10-CM allows for the capture of information regarding risk factors to health, such as lifestyle, life management, psychosocial circumstances, and occupational or physical environment.

Advantages to more detailed diagnosis coding include:
- reducing requests for additional documentation to support claims for medical necessity;
- allowing the capture of accurate data on new ways of describing diseases due to advances in medicine;
- providing data to support performance measurement, outcomes analysis, cost analysis, and monitoring resource utilization; and
- increasing the sensitivity of the classification when refinements are made in applications, such as grouping methods.

How can we ensure that the documentation will be sufficient when ICD-10-CM is implemented? As stated earlier, an ICD-10-CM readiness audit provides the ability to identify the problem areas, and this will help practices formulate documentation and training needs for practitioners.

It is beneficial to begin this process now by reviewing five or six records per week for each practitioner. Keep in mind that only the diagnoses are assessed for this audit to prepare for ICD-10-CM. In order to conduct the audit, the auditor must have the ICD-10-CM codes, guidelines, and indices, in addition to a current ICD-9-CM code book.

The ICD-10-CM codes are available at no charge on the CMS Web site at www.cms.hhs.gov/ICD10. The Tabular List and Alphabetic Index, along with the GEMs (described later in this chapter) and the Table of Drugs and Chemicals, are also available on this Web site. It would be helpful for every practice to have a copy of this information.

Review Figure 4.10, which is an illustration of what an audit report might look like.

FIGURE 4.10 Sample Audit Report

PHYSICIAN NAME: Family Practice, MD   **DATE OF AUDIT:** 10/20/200x

REVIEWER (AUDITOR): Jane Doe, CPC, CPC-H, CCS-P

Chart	Patient ID	Documented Diagnosis (description)	ICD-9-CM Diagnosis Documented	ICD-10-CM Diagnosis Documented	
1	0398M	Gastroesophageal reflux (GERD)	530.81	K21 K21.0	Gastroesophageal reflux Gastroesophageal reflux disease with esophagitis
				K21.9	Gastroesophageal reflux disease without esophagitis
2	0519F	Diaper rash	691.10	L22	Diaper dermatitis Diaper rash

Note that, with patient 0398M, GERD is coded 530.81 in ICD-9-CM, but in ICD-10-CM more information is required. The user needs more information, such as whether the GERD is with or without esophagitis.

When a month of weekly audits has been completed and results compiled, it is beneficial to review with the provider the chart note with the documented ICD-9-CM code versus the ICD-10-CM code (if it can be coded). One major issue, in many cases, is that it may not be possible to assign the more appropriate diagnosis code in ICD-10-CM because of the lack of documented specificity in the medical record.

As can be seen in the sample audit report, only one of the medical records reviewed might support ICD-10-CM coding. The encounter for the gastroesophageal reflux would need more information in order to report the diagnosis code accurately.

How is the problem of the lack of documentation solved?

IMPLEMENTATION TIP

Reviewing five or six records per week for diagnosis deficiencies will help improve diagnosis specificity for ICD-10-CM.

- Educate physicians by showing them the comparison between both coding systems.
- Encourage practitioners to begin documenting more specifically for ICD-10-CM.
- Keep results each week and compile a monthly summary. This summary should identify the percentage of correct documentation for both ICD-9-CM and ICD-10-CM with a recommendation for improving documentation.

IMPLEMENTATION TIP

Be sure to approach the documentation improvement work as a collaborative effort between the auditor and the clinical staff. If the work is perceived as being punitive, it will hamper the improvement process.

The most important mechanisms in working with physician documentation issues are communication, communication, and communication. If the physician can see where documentation improvements are needed by reviewing the medical record along with the audit results, it will provide a clearer picture of the impact documentation has on ICD-10-CM coding.

It will be evident after documentation is reviewed that a lot of work must be completed to get ready for ICD-10-CM. The practitioner's diagnosis documentation should be audited for approximately 6 to 12 months or until ICD-10-CM is implemented. Areas that need improvement should be tracked on a spreadsheet and shared with the practice. Be sure that examples of documentation shared within the practice do not identify the individual patient or practitioner. Tracking documentation issues will help identify education needs for the practice. Identifying "target risk" areas in the practice will promote discussion and resolution for the implementation project team. Develop the project strategy for documentation improvement.

Step 6: Develop a Communication Plan

It is important to get everyone in the practice involved in the implementation project by informing all staff as to the reasons for moving to ICD-10-CM, what time frame is necessary for implementation, and how ICD-10-CM will affect the practice. First, develop materials to disseminate to managers and staff regarding the timeline and status of implementation. Communication might include staff meetings, newsletters, e-mails, or other methods of communication. A schedule should also be developed for when the information will be communicated.

Staff members need to understand not just what is happening but what they need to do and how it will impact their work. By communicating this information during the early phase of implementation, managers can make staff members aware of their responsibilities and roles in the implementation process. Training schedules and training plans should be communicated to staff early to avoid causing them anxiety about learning ICD-10-CM. It is beneficial to conduct periodic briefings for staff to keep the entire practice updated on the progress of the project.

Step 7: Develop a Training Plan

A critical step for the implementation of ICD-10-CM is the development of a comprehensive, effective training program. Development and implementation of a training plan can take two or more years. Preparation of an education plan for ICD-10-CM might sound easy, but think about the impact of the training on the practice. A "buy in" from the entire practice is necessary to accomplish a successful training plan. The time to begin planning is not three months prior to the implementation deadline. The time to begin is now.

The following are recommended steps to take in developing a training plan:

1 Define training objectives

2 Assess baseline training needs

3 Identify training media

4 Provide training

5 Measure effectiveness of training.

Define Training Objectives

The overall goal of training will be to have all staff involved with identification and coding trained on ICD-10-CM and associated workflow process changes at the time ICD-10-CM is implemented, so that normal business operations and billing continue without interruptions.

To meet the overall goal, a training timeline should be developed to identify milestones that need to be reached, and these should be correctly sequenced so that the goal can be achieved. Milestones within the training plan include assessing baseline knowledge, providing training, and measuring outcomes of training.

Assess Baseline Training Needs

Begin the assessment by identifying which staff members in the practice need to be trained on ICD-10-CM. Next, analyze how detailed the training will need to be for those individuals. The amount of training will depend on each person's role in the practice. Staff directly involved in the billing and revenue cycle will need the most intensive training on ICD-10-CM. Clinical staff training will need to be focused on the impact documentation will have on the ability to code.

Assessment should be made of staff members' knowledge of anatomy, physiology, pharmacology (medications), and medical terminology. Keep in mind that ICD-10-CM has a higher level of detail than ICD-9-CM and will require an expanded knowledge of these key areas. Staff who have a working knowledge of anatomy and physiology will have a shorter time span for training, a shorter learning curve, and increased competency with ICD-10-CM. It is important before the training plan is begun to evaluate internal competencies to determine whether to provide training internally or to contract for services from outside professionals.

There are many resources on the Internet for testing skill sets. There are even some free Web sites that allow the user to review medical terminology and anatomy and complete a short test to assess understanding. The University of Minnesota offers free testing for anatomy on its Web site: http://msjensen.cehd. umn.edu/webanatomy. There are other Web sites, such as *Universal Class*. This group charges a fee for courses, but the fees are affordable. Their Web site can be accessed at: www.universalclass.com/i/crn/30444.htm. There are more than 900,000 online sites for anatomy and medical terminology. Here are a few other Web sites that might be useful:

- www.corexcel.com/html/online.medical.terminology.htm
- www.expertrating.com/awareness-tests/Anatomy-Terminology-Certification.asp
- www.becomehealthynow.com/article/bodycell/709/2/
- www.ritecode.com/.

The American Academy of Professional Coders and the American Health Information Management Association (AHIMA) have several online courses for anatomy, terminology, pathophysiology, and pharmacology as well as seminars and workshops that can help a practice prepare for ICD-10-CM. The information can be accessed on the AAPC Web site at: www.aapc.com. The AHIMA Web site is: www.ahima.org.

Training on ICD-10-CM will have to be individualized on the basis of the staff members' roles in their practices and their current knowledge of diagnosis coding. Keep in mind that training must also address any practice workflow changes that will be made as a result of implementing ICD-10-CM.

Next, consider how much time each staff member will need for training. Determining how much training various staff members need can be based on informal assessments, such as considering members' roles in the practice and their overall knowledge levels. Again, billing staff will need the most time to learn the ICD-10-CM coding structure and any work processes that will change as a result of the implementation.

Specifically for medical coders in the practice, measurement of their baseline knowledge of anatomy, physiology, medication, and medical terminology must be conducted, and their knowledge must be enhanced and/or updated as needed to prepare them for the higher level of detail in ICD-10-CM. This process can take up to one year and is critical for laying a solid foundation for ICD-10-CM. Ensuring that coders' baseline knowledge is at the appropriate level will ultimately shorten the learning curve and reduce the level of degradation of medical knowledge while lessening anticipated backlogs and speeding the realization of benefits from ICD-10-CM.

Find out how the staff learns best. Some people are visual learners and need an instructor for help and guidance, whereas others learn well using self-study or e-learning as the preferred method. In many cases, a combination of classroom/seminar and self-study or e-learning is appropriate.

The timing of training should also be customized to the staff members and their roles in the practice. Experience has shown that staff trained too early in the process will have forgotten much of the information by the time of the final implementation date. If staff are trained too late, they may be overwhelmed by the training and final steps of the system implementation occurring at the same time. The exact timing of training will depend on the practice and the experience level of the staff. Approximately six to nine months prior to the go-live date is considered to be an appropriate window for optimal staff training.

Identify Training Media

The training process might take up to one year or more to complete, depending on budgets, resources available, and size of the practice. From the baseline assessment, the project team will have an understanding of how detailed the training will need to be and whether or not to include additional topics, such as anatomy, physiology, medication, and medical terminology. The team will also have a better understanding of how much time staff will need for training and how they will best learn.

Begin by identifying training resources readily accessible to the practice. Are they available online? Are there onsite training programs being held in the area? What books and written materials are available for the specialty of the practice? The project team will want to review the costs of the various training media and compare this with the amount budgeted for training.

There are many exceptional training opportunities through various organizations. As the compliance date for ICD-10-CM moves closer, there will likely be increases in the number and types of educational opportunities, including:

- audio seminars;
- convention presentations;
- local conference and chapter presentations from various organizations;
- online training; and
- workshops and seminars.

It might be beneficial to obtain a self-study training module on ICD-10-CM guidelines, which might include a self-test at the end of the module. Consider attending a workshop, seminar, or course on ICD-10-CM. There are many ICD-10-CM courses available right now, and many more will be available as the implementation deadline approaches.

What about a classroom model? If the practice is primary care or a specialty that typically uses many diagnosis codes, a classroom, seminar, or online course might be more beneficial. Courses based on specialty will become more common as ICD-10-CM implementation moves forward. Consider a combination of e-learning, self-study, and classroom learning to accomplish the training goal.

Keep in mind that the front office staff, managers, and clinical and ancillary staff may not need the extensive training that physicians, nonphysician providers, coders, and billers will need. The front office staff, managers, and clinical and ancillary staff might need 6 to 10 hours of training on average. A seminar or e-learning environment might be a good avenue for this group, provided that the training is related to the specialty. A seminar that is too generic has little benefit. A seminar to review ICD-10-CM guidelines is fine to start preparation, but a specialty-specific session for understanding of specific ICD-10-CM chapters that will be used day to day in the practice may also be useful.

Physicians, coders, and nonphysician practitioners might benefit from participating in a full course or having an instructor (internal or external) plan a curriculum over several months to cover all avenues of ICD-10-CM coding. Use real case studies specific to the specialty, so the training makes sense to the providers and coders. A post-test is useful for determining whether participants understand ICD-10-CM coding concepts.

The project team will want to have resources available within the practice to support staff after they complete their training and begin implementing ICD-10-CM. These resources may be the print materials obtained from seminars and on-line courses as well as other books or newsletters.

Once the training approach has been decided, the project team will need to finalize the sources of the training. If the practice decides to provide training using a course or workshop, will it be conducted using internal or external sources? Is there someone in the practice who is ICD-10-CM coding savvy? Can one staff person obtain the training and then train the rest of the staff? This may be a good approach for smaller practices with limited resources.

If the practice does not have the time to prepare and deliver training, consider external sources. Contract with an instructor, consultant, or other organization that can deliver the training over a specified period. Seminars are good adjunctive training options, but staff cannot really learn ICD-10-CM in one day.

Provide Training

The next step is for staff to undergo the actual training. Again, keep in mind the timing of when the training occurs in relation to the implementation deadline. Staff members need to be properly prepared when the compliance date arrives. Advance preparation will make the training and the transition much smoother.

It might be beneficial to split the training into two phases—the first phase for the overview of ICD-10-CM and the second phase for more in-depth training, including the code set and guidelines. A practice might think of the transition to ICD-10-CM like the preparations necessary for implementation of the Health Insurance Portability and Accountability Act. If the practice was prepared well in advance, the process was easier to accomplish. Practices should allow, at minimum, a year to complete training for the entire group.

Information obtained in one-day training sessions, in most cases, is not retained for a sufficiently long period for persons who will be using ICD-10-CM on a day-to-day basis. Keep in mind that documentation issues should be addressed in any training with providers. Reinforce the importance of specificity required in ICD-10-CM and that documentation is the key. As part of a training plan six to twelve months prior to implementation, formulate a training schedule. For example, one year prior to implementation, the project team might focus on e-learning, audio conferences, and seminars to get ready for ICD-10-CM. Four to six months prior to implementation, the training should be more in-depth, so everyone has a good understanding of ICD-10-CM.

Either within the training or separately within the practice, the staff should be educated on the benefits and value of ICD-10-CM, particularly within the context of national health care data quality and the improvement in the quality of care with ICD-10-CM coding. Everyone should understand the regulatory process for adoption, the compliance timeline, and the variables that may affect the timeline for adoption. Staff should understand how ICD-10-CM will evolve with the EMR and the national health information infrastructure. Many valuable resources are listed in Appendix C of this publication.

The project team should also map out when the training will occur for each staff person. Pay particular attention to who will be at the training to ensure there is enough staff to continue practice operations during that time. If the practice is unable to stagger the training or if a large percentage of the staff need to attend offsite training, the project team can plan ahead for patient scheduling for that time.

Another consideration is whether to hire temporary staff to support the practice's business operations during the training period. Temporary staff may be needed only for key positions in the practice and for a specified number of days. Be sure to factor into the budget the expense of temporary staff.

Measure Effectiveness of Training

Once training is completed, the project team will want to determine how effective the training was. One suggestion is to have the coders and/or providers begin using ICD-10-CM along with ICD-9-CM simultaneously six months to a year prior to implementation. This will assist the practice to re-evaluate documentation areas for improvement and the amount of time it takes to code with ICD-10-CM. Keep in mind that there is a learning curve, and productivity might be compromised for a short period. However, with diligence in planning and training, the coders and providers will become comfortable with ICD-10-CM, which will increase productivity.

The project team will also want to determine whether the coders and providers have developed the necessary level of proficiency. One way to measure training success is to perform an audit of the test medical records that have been coded using ICD-10-CM. Another way to measure whether the training was successful is to provide a test a few weeks after training to measure retention. Both methods will be useful in identifying weaknesses in coding and/or documentation that can be corrected prior to going live with ICD-10-CM.

It is a good idea to measure the coders' and providers' understanding of ICD-10-CM at one to three months prior to implementation and to provide customized learning to fill any knowledge deficits. This will also be a good time to formulate new policies and procedures as part of the practice compliance plan. Communication will be important in making staff comfortable with ICD-10-CM and can take their newly developed skills beyond implementation.

Training is a vital part of ensuring success with ICD-10-CM. A well-defined training plan will benefit the entire implementation process. Review the ICD-10-CM training development map example in Figure 4.11.

> **IMPLEMENTATION TIP**
>
> Once training is completed, testing and outcomes measurement will validate users' understanding of ICD-10-CM coding.

FIGURE 4.11 **ICD-10-CM Training Development Map**

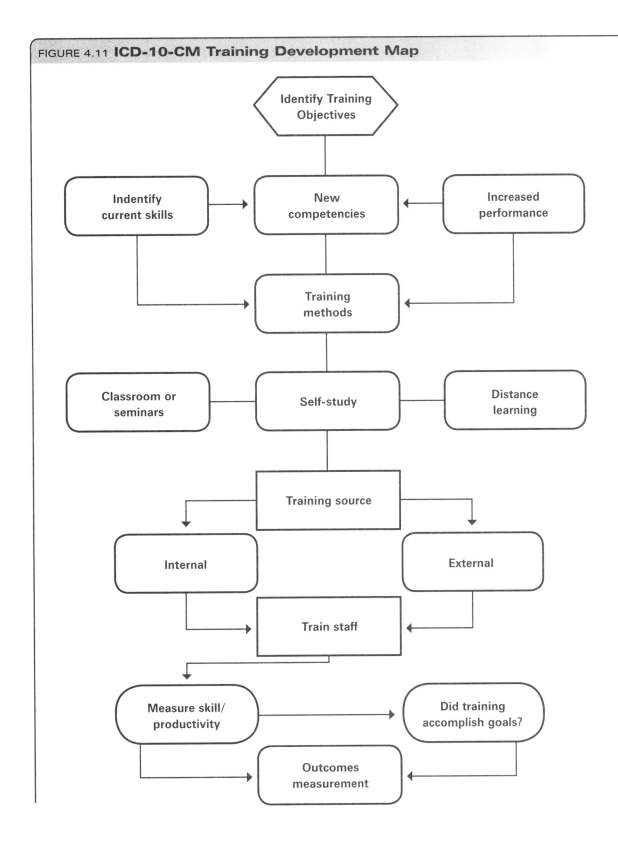

Step 8: Complete Information System Design and Development

The next step in the implementation process, which is to work with system vendors regarding upgrades from ICD-9-CM to ICD-10-CM, should begin at least one year prior to the ICD-10-CM compliance date. However, begin talking to system vendors two years prior to implementation. Whatever type of practice management or information system the practice uses, structural changes are inherent to ICD-10-CM, and upgrades must be made to the system. Multiple code sets, including ICD-9-CM, ICD-10-CM, Current Procedural Terminology, and the Healthcare Common Procedural Coding System, must be supported in the system upgrade. Changing code sets will involve more than expansion of the field definition to seven characters in the databases where the procedure codes and diagnosis codes are stored, although that will be part of the process. Program logic that depends on the diagnosis will need revision. Areas that might be impacted include the following:

- Programs
- Screens
- Documentation
- Forms (electronic and printed).

In addition, software applications for abstraction of coding data, utilization management tools, claims editors, billing software, data reporting tools, coding edits, groupers, and clinical systems must be revised. Every electronic transaction that requires ICD-9-CM needs to accommodate ICD-10-CM.

The project team will also want to consider storage requirements. Hardware and disk space will need to be increased to accommodate the larger classification schemes. Because ICD-10-CM is much larger than ICD-9-CM, fields will need to be modified within the system to accommodate the alphanumeric codes. Both ICD-9-CM and ICD-10-CM will need to be supported, because unpaid claims might still be outstanding for a period of time after implementation.

Practices are even more diverse than hospitals, ranging from large, multispecialty organizations with multiple locations to solo practitioners. At the upper end, a large practice may have a range of systems similar to that of a large hospital, including financial, clinical, medical management, and billing systems. These organizations may have a mix of purchased systems from multiple vendors and in-house legacy systems with multiple interfaces between internal systems and with external business partners.

Updating particular software packages is only one part of the process. Most large practices have multiple systems and exchange data with outside organizations. The interfaces between internal systems and business partners must be revised to accommodate ICD-10-CM, as must any electronic transactions using diagnostic or procedure codes.

Existing data must be converted, and provisions must be made to support both ICD-9-CM and ICD-10-CM, or parallel systems must be maintained during a transition period. The most efficient approach will vary. Reports, whether on-line or hard copy, will also need to be reformatted and in some cases restructured. Similarly, paper forms and the work flows will also need to be revised or redesigned.

The extent of the conversion will depend on the number of computer systems in place, whether those systems are purchased or developed in-house, the age and flexibility of each system, the number of internal system interfaces and reports, and the number of external data transfers and reports to business partners and other entities.

Most practices now have automated billing and scheduling systems and are in the process of implementing even more sophisticated systems, such as EMRs, electronic prescribing systems, and clinical ordering systems. Larger practices tend to be further along in adopting health information technology. The information systems of some solo practitioners may be limited to a desktop computer with the minimum amount of purchased software necessary to support billing. In this case, the implementation may be limited to the installation and testing of updated software from a single vendor, conversion of existing data or parallel operation of two versions for a time, and purchasing revised paper forms.

Implementation involving the information system depends on the size of the practice and the type of systems in place. The larger practice will incur higher costs and more complex conversion than a small solo practice that uses one or two desktop computers with a practice management system. The more complex the systems in place, the more costly the conversion will be.

Data Mapping

Data mapping or code mapping is an attempt to translate equivalent meaning from source to target. For example, if a diagnosis code is being mapped from ICD-9-CM to a code in ICD-10-CM, the source is the ICD-9-CM code, and the target is the code it is being mapped to (ICD-10-CM). One source-system code is linked to one or more target-system codes. To enable data reporting during and after the ICD-10-CM transition, code data maps are needed. Codes will need to be mapped in two ways:

- Forward mapping from ICD-9-CM to ICD-10-CM
- Backward mapping from ICD-10-CM to ICD-9-CM.

Mapping will be used to test and convert systems, link data, develop application-specific mappings, and analyze data collection during the transition period and most likely beyond implementation.

Figure 4.12 is an example of code mapping for acute pharyngitis from ICD-9-CM (source) to ICD-10-CM (target).

FIGURE 4.12 **GEMs Mapping, Acute Pharyngitis**	
ICD-9-CM Code	**ICD-10-CM Code**
462 Acute pharyngitis	J02 Acute pharyngitis
	J02.0 Streptococcal pharyngitis
	J02.8 Acute pharyngitis due to other specified organism
	J02.9 Acute pharyngitis, unspecified

Notice in Figure 4.12 that the ICD-9-CM code for acute pharyngitis maps to three codes in ICD-10-CM. The ICD-10-CM codes are more specific than those in ICD-9-CM, and more specific information will be needed. Mapping will be an important step for information systems as well as internally in the practice.

GEMs is a system developed to map ICD-9-CM to ICD-10-CM. This method has two GEMs files, with each file containing code pairs—one code pair from each set. The first file is a mapping of the ICD-10-CM codes to the ICD-9-CM codes, and the second file is a mapping from ICD-9-CM codes to the ICD-10-CM codes. Specific flags are additional information useful to mapping.

These files are reference mapping for the health care industry that uses coded data. GEMs are more than just a map. GEMs are a two-way translation dictionary for diagnosis codes from which maps can be developed. The files can be easily converted into a spreadsheet or database to assist with mapping the diagnosis codes in a practice. The GEMs files have a PDF user's guide for help in how to use the system. This system will be discussed in greater detail in Chapter 8.

GEMs were developed as a coordinated effort with the National Center for Health Statistics, the American Hospital Association, AHIMA, and CMS. These files are reference mappings that are in the public domain, which means anyone can use them. The files are located on the CMS Web site at www.cms.hhs.gov/ICD10.

Figure 4.13 is an illustration of a sample workflow for a medium-sized practice with 10 physicians and staff.

Step 9: Conduct a Business Process Analysis

Once a practice has an understanding of ICD-10-CM and how it operates, an analysis of how its use will impact the business processes is necessary. It could take several months to conduct this analysis. Conduct a detailed review of the practice to determine the process of how ICD-9-CM is currently used (ie, Superbills or EMRs).

Another issue to consider is a review of health plan contracts and billing procedures. It is possible that health plans will modify contracts as a result of the move to ICD-10-CM. Most health plan policies list diagnosis codes that support medical necessity for certain services. A review of the policies that are applicable to the specialty will be useful in avoiding claim denials after implementation. Because of the greater specificity in the ICD-10-CM codes, the health plan might better recognize the severity of patients' conditions and could adjust payment schedules according to the clinical condition. Although procedure coding

IMPLEMENTATION TIP

Updating software may not be the only process in the practice. Make sure hardware and disk space will be able to accommodate ICD-10-CM.

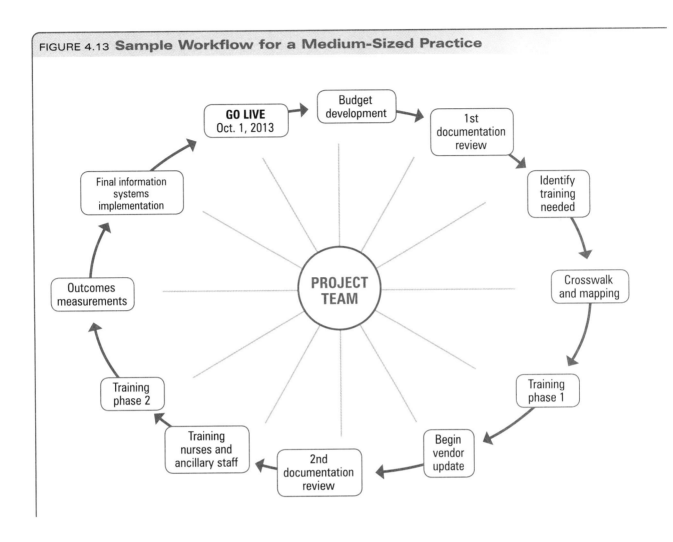

FIGURE 4.13 **Sample Workflow for a Medium-Sized Practice**

will not change for physician practice or outpatient facilities, the impact of ICD-10-CM on payment is currently unknown. Diagnosis codes might also be used for medical review, auditing, and coverage determination.

Analyze how the change to ICD-10-CM will impact the patient and overall patient care in the practice. Will the change reduce the number of patients the physician treats per day? Will more claim denials resulting from lack of supporting medical necessity, on the basis of health plan policy, impact the patient and the practice? Will there be a delay in receiving reimbursement after implementation because of system problems? Does the practice have sufficient funds to handle a delay in cash flow? If a practice is small and does not have the staff to conduct the analysis, an outside consulting firm should be hired to assist with the project. This project could take three to four months, depending on the scope of the analysis and the size of the practice.

Step 10: Conduct a Needs Assessment

What other tools will the practice need? If the practice currently does not have a coding look-up program, or in a larger practice an "encoder," it might be time to invest in one of these tools. The practice might also consider a conversion to an EMR system during the transition. EMRs can assist in coding but should not be used for that purpose only. Coders will still be needed to review the EMR documentation to ensure that it supports the service the physician reports on the claim. Other tools that might be useful for the staff are anatomy books, additional coding reference materials (electronic and paper format), and an upgrade to the hardware system.

On February 17, 2009, the American Recovery and Reinvestment Act was signed into law. The health information technology component of the Bill, the HITECH Act, appropriates $19.2 billion to encourage the adoption of electronic health records.

As a result of this legislation, the Congressional Budget Office estimates that approximately 90% of doctors and 70% of hospitals will be using comprehensive electronic health records within the next decade. This legislation provides immediate funding for health information technology infrastructure, training, dissemination of best practices, telemedicine, inclusion of health information technology in clinical education, and state grants to promote health information technology.

In addition, the legislation provides significant financial incentives through the Medicare and Medicaid programs to encourage doctors and hospitals to adopt and use certified electronic health records. Physicians will be eligible for $40,000 to $65,000 for showing that they are meaningfully using health information technology, such as through the reporting of quality measures. Federally qualified health centers, rural health clinics, children's hospitals and others will be eligible for funding through the Medicaid program.

Incentive payments for both physicians and hospitals will continue for several years but will be phased out over time. Eventually, Medicare payments will be reduced for physicians who do not use certified electronic health records that allow them to electronically communicate with others.

The legislation also provides additional funds to states for low-interest loans to help providers finance health information technology and grants to regional health information exchanges to unite local providers. Grants are also offered for the development and adoption of electronic health records for providers other than physicians and hospitals.

Step 11: Complete Deployment of the System Changes

Testing of the information system(s) should begin no later than the first quarter of 2013. The project team (or a biller) will want to test all of the transactions that use ICD-10-CM. To test the transactions, contact trading partners (clearinghouses and health plans) to set up a schedule of when transactions can be sent to them. A practice will want to test with as many of its trading partners as possible. The project team should focus on the trading partners and transactions that make up the highest percentage of practice revenue and overall volume. The team will need to budget for the additional time and expense of conducting the testing. Once the testing is complete, it is important to review the results to identify what worked and what changes still need to be addressed. Testing with trading partners is the best opportunity a practice will have to make certain that the ICD-10-CM codes will be received and interpreted properly after the compliance deadline.

Once the information systems are converted, a documentation improvement phase has been done, and training is completed, the effectiveness of the training should be evaluated to ensure all staff are ready for the compliance date. Identify specific metrics that are needed to assess performance using ICD-10-CM. Metrics may include internal audits of documentation compared to coding, comparisons of the number of delayed or pending claims under ICD-9-CM versus ICD-10-CM, and comparisons of reimbursement for services under ICD-9-CM versus ICD-10-CM.

Following implementation, refresher training might be beneficial for the staff. It will provide an opportunity to assess staff members' understanding of ICD-10-CM and any new workflow processes. Also, additional overtime might be necessary to follow up on delayed or denied claims and/or system problems. It might be useful for small or medium-sized practices to have vendor and outside consulting assistance for the first few months after implementation to troubleshoot problems that might occur.

Summary

Making the transition to ICD-10-CM will require commitment from the practice. Some organizations, such as large hospitals, plan to spend the first year on system readiness and the second year on training. The decision on how implementation is done is up to the practice.

Some steps to ease the transition to ICD-10 include the following.

- Begin by identifying a project team to assist in the planning and implementation of ICD-10-CM. This is important even for solo practitioners.
- Create a timeline to identify steps and priorities early.
- Budget for ICD-10-CM implementation accurately. Research actual costs based on practice needs and previous experience with changes of this scale.
- Begin the transition process now.
- Allow for adequate time for migration and training.
- Use an outside consultant if staff resources are limited or for expert assistance from an outside source.
- Talk to system vendors early. Find out whether they are preparing for ICD-10-CM and will be able to accommodate the new coding system.
- Develop a training plan for practitioners, clinical staff, coders/billers, and other ancillary staff, based on the types of duties they perform.
- Implement training in phases, keeping in mind that if training is conducted too early, retention may be lost, and if it is started too late it may cause additional confusion in the practice.
- Review health plan contracts and medical policy to determine how the practice will be affected.
- Monitor ICD-10-CM implementation progress in the practice by communicating with all parties and keeping the entire practice informed.

- Test system readiness prior to implementation.
- Continuously assess the progress of the implementation at each step. Ongoing feedback will identify what is going well and what areas need additional effort.

By planning ahead, using the talent and resources in the practice, and keeping up on the legislative progress on ICD-10-CM, a practice will afford a fairly smooth transition to ICD-10-CM.

Resources

Libicki M, Brahmakulam, I. RAND Science and Technology. *The Costs and Benefits of Moving to the ICD-10 Code Sets.* Available online at www.rand.org/pubs/technical_reports/2004/RAND_TR132.pdf.

The Nolan Study. Examining the Cost of Implementing ICD-10; The Hay Group

Centers for Medicare & Medicaid Services, 2008. *ICD-10-CM, July 2007 release.* Available online at www.cms.hhs.gov/ICD10.

General Equivalency Mapping Files. Available online at www.cms.hhs.gov/ICD10/downloads/reimb_map_guide_2009.pdf.

Nachimson Advisors, LLC. *The Impact of Implementing ICD-10 on Physician Practices and Clinical Laboratories: A Report to the ICD10 Coalition.* Available online at http://nachimsonadvisors.com/Documents/ICD-10%20 Impacts%20on%20Providers.pdf.

The American Recovery and Reinvestment Act of 2009. Available online at http://frwebgate.access.gpo.gov/cgi-bin/getdoc.cgi?dbname=111_cong_bills&docid=f:h1enr.pdf.

End-of-Chapter Questions

1   Name the five recommended steps for ICD-10-CM implementation
    in the practice.

    a. _____

    b. _____

    c. _____

    d. _____

    e. _____

2   For budgeting, what is the average dollar amount that a practice
    might spend on system upgrades? _____

3   When a budget is created, what other expenditures besides system
    upgrades need to be considered? _____

4   Why is a documentation review/audit beneficial for preparation for
    ICD-10-CM implementation? _____

5   List the six types of training media available today.

    a. _____

    b. _____

    c. _____

    d. _____

    e. _____

    f. _____

CHAPTER 5

Format and Structure of ICD-10-CM

OBJECTIVES

- Understand the similarities and differences in the structure and format of the International Classification of Diseases, Tenth Revision, Clinical Modification (ICD-10-CM)
- Review categories or "blocks" in ICD-10-CM
- Review the conventions in ICD-10-CM
- Understand the fifth to seventh character extensions
- Understand the use of dummy placeholders

Introduction

This chapter will cover the conventions and format of ICD-10-CM, along with specific category characteristics of ICD-10-CM. The process of converting from ICD-9-CM to ICD-10-CM affects many aspects of the health care system, including revision of instruction manuals and medical software as well as information technology systems and other coding tools used in medical practices. A good general understanding of ICD-10-CM is beneficial for all practices while they prepare for implementation.

As stated in Chapter 1, ICD-10-CM is similar to ICD-9-CM in that some terminology, conventions, classifications, and other features are similar. This chapter will cover the ICD-10-CM basic information that every user will need in order to successfully use ICD-10-CM. There are notable improvements in the content and format of ICD-10-CM, which include:

- the addition of information relevant to ambulatory and managed care encounters;
- expanded injury codes in which ICD-10-CM groups injuries by site of the injury, as opposed to grouping in ICD-9-CM by type of injury or type of wound;
- creation of combination diagnosis/symptom codes, which reduces the number of codes needed to fully describe a condition;
- greater specificity in code assignment;
- V and E codes being incorporated into the main classification in ICD-10-CM;
- ICD-10-CM codes being alphanumeric and including all letters except U;
- the length of codes in ICD-10-CM being a maximum of seven characters, as opposed to five digits in ICD-9-CM; and
- some vacant, three-character categories in ICD-10-CM to allow for revisions/future expansion.

Classification

A classification is a method of grouping according to *purpose* and codifying with numerical (or alphanumerical) identification according to certain principles. A statistical classification can allow for different levels of detail if it has a hierarchical structure with subdivisions. A statistical classification of diseases should retain the ability both to identify specific disease entities and to allow statistical presentation of data for broader groups to enable obtaining useful and understandable information.

A classification of diseases can be defined as a system of categories to which morbid entities are assigned according to established criteria. ICD-10-CM is used to translate diagnoses of diseases and other health problems from words into an alphanumeric code, which permits easy storage, retrieval, and analysis of the data.

ICD-10 represents the International Statistical Classification of Diseases and Related Health Problems. ICD-10-CM is used to classify data recorded under headings such as diagnosis, reason for admission, conditions treated, and reason for consultation that appear on a wide variety of health records and from which statistics and other health information are derived.

ICD-10-CM will add many more code choices. The first character is alphabetic, so instead of 10 choices, there may be up to 26 choices. The specificity of the codes encompasses up to seven character extensions with dummy placeholders to allow room for expansion. The ICD-10-CM classification system contains 21 chapters and has supplementary classification chapters. In comparison, ICD-9-CM has only 17 chapters and two supplementary chapters for V codes and E codes.

In Chapters 6 through 8 of this book, the general and chapter-specific guidelines will be reviewed. Further guidance on the use of the classification may be found in the Official Coding and Reporting Guidelines section of ICD-10-CM, available at ftp://ftp.cdc.gov/pub/Health_Statistics/NCHS/Publications/ICD10CM/2009/.

ICD-10 is copyrighted by the World Health Organization and reproduced by permission for US government purposes. The guidelines and codes may also be found on the National Center for Health Statistics Web site at www.cdc.gov/nchs.

Many of the symbols, terminology, and conventions from ICD-9-CM are carried forward in ICD-10-CM, which will help make the conversion easier.

ICD-10-CM far exceeds its predecessors in the number of codes available. The disease classification has been expanded to include health-related conditions and to provide greater specificity at the six-digit level and with a seventh digit extension. The sixth and seventh characters are not optional; they are intended for use in recording the information documented in the medical record.

Comparison of ICD-9-CM to ICD-10-CM

ICD-9-CM has 17 chapters, compared with 21 chapters in ICD-10-CM, which includes separate chapters for the eye and adnexa and the ear. The chapters are subdivided into blocks of three alphanumeric character categories. In addition, the classifications *External Cause of Morbidity and Mortality* and *Factors Influencing Health Status and Contact with Health Services* (V and E codes in ICD-9-CM) are not considered supplemental classifications in ICD-10-CM and have their own chapter classifications (Chapters 20 and 21).

Table 5.1 is a comparison of chapter numbers and titles in ICD-9-CM to those in ICD-10-CM. Notice that Diseases of the Eye and Adnexa and Diseases of the Ear and Mastoid Process will have their own chapters in ICD-10-CM.

TABLE 5.1 **Comparison of Chapter Numbers and Titles in ICD-9-CM to Those in ICD-10-CM**

Chapter	ICD-9-CM	ICD-10-CM
1	Infectious and Parasitic Diseases	Certain Infectious and Parasitic Diseases
2	Neoplasms	Malignant Neoplasms
3	Endocrine, Nutritional and Metabolic Diseases, and Immunity Disorders	Disease of the Blood and Blood-Forming Organs and Certain Disorders involving Immune Mechanism
4	Diseases of the Blood and Blood-Forming Organs	Endocrine, Nutritional and Metabolic Diseases
5	Mental Disorders	Mental and Behavioral Disorders
6	Diseases of the Nervous System and Sense Organs	Diseases of the Nervous System
7	Diseases of the Circulatory System	Diseases of the Eye and Adnexa
8	Diseases of the Respiratory System	Diseases of the Ear and Mastoid Process
9	Diseases of the Digestive System	Diseases of the Circulatory System
10	Diseases of the Genitourinary System	Diseases of the Respiratory System
11	Complications of Pregnancy, Childbirth, and the Puerperium	Diseases of the Digestive System
12	Diseases of the Skin and Subcutaneous Tissue	Diseases of the Skin and Subcutaneous Tissue

	TABLE 5.1 **Comparison of Chapter Numbers and Titles in ICD-9-CM to Those in ICD-10-CM** *(continued)*	
Chapter	**ICD-9-CM**	**ICD-10-CM**
13	Diseases of the Musculoskeletal System and Connective Tissue	Diseases of the Musculoskeletal System and Connective Tissue
14	Congenital Anomalies	Diseases of the Genitourinary System
15	Certain Conditions Originating in the Perinatal Period	Pregnancy, Childbirth, and the Puerperium
16	Symptoms, Signs, and Ill-Defined Conditions	Certain Conditions Originating in the Newborn (Perinatal) Period
17	Injury and Poisoning	Congenital Malformations, Deformations, and Chromosomal Abnormalities
18	N/A	Symptoms, Signs, and Abnormal Clinical and Laboratory Findings, Not Elsewhere Classified
19	N/A	Injury, Poisoning, and Certain Other Consequences of External Causes
20	N/A	External Causes of Morbidity
21	N/A	Factors Influencing Health Status and Contact with Health Services
Supplementary classification	Classification of Factors Influencing Health Status and Contact with Health Services (V codes)	N/A
Supplementary classification	Classification of External Cause of Injury and Poisoning (E Codes)	N/A

Chapters in ICD-10-CM will be similar to those of ICD-9-CM. The differences are the following:

- Alphanumeric structure
- Addition of six-digit and seven-digit extensions to provide a higher level of specificity
- More specificity
- Reorganization and addition of chapters
- More precise diagnostic codes
- Expansion to include health-related conditions
- Creation of combination diagnosis/symptom codes to reduce the number of codes needed to fully describe a condition.

ICD-10-CM Characteristics and Structure

ICD-10-CM consists of the following:

- Tabular lists containing cause-of-death titles and codes (Volume 1)
- Inclusion and exclusion terms for cause-of-death titles (Volume 1)
- Alphabetic Index to diseases and nature of injury
- External Causes of Injury
- Table of Drugs and Chemicals (Volume 3)
- Description, Guidelines, and Coding Rules (Volume 2).

ICD-10-CM is divided into the Alphabetic Index, which is an alphabetic list of terms and their corresponding codes, and the Tabular List, a numerical list of codes divided by chapter, according to condition or body system.

Alphabetic Index

ICD-10-CM is similar to ICD-9-CM as it uses an indented format for ease of reference. The Alphabetic Index (Volume 2) is organized in the same manner as in ICD-9-CM. Codes are listed by a main term, which describes the disease and/or condition. As in ICD-9-CM, there are exceptions to the rule.

Cross-references such as *see* and *see also* are found in ICD-10-CM. Notes appear in the Alphabetic Index to:

- define terms;
- provide direction; and
- provide coding instructions.

The structure of the Alphabetic Index is similar to that of ICD-9-CM. The index provides separate sections to access terms related to:

- disorders;
- diseases;
- poisonings;
- adverse effects;
- external causes; and
- conditions.

The Alphabetic Index is divided into three sections:

1   Terms from Chapters 1 through 19 and Chapter 21 and the Table of Neoplasms

2   Terms related to external causes of morbidity and Chapter 20 terms

3   Table of Drugs and Chemicals.

As in ICD-9-CM, the Alphabetic Index in ICD-10-CM is organized in bold type by main term. Subordinate terms and modifiers are located under the main terms, following an indented format. Nonessential modifiers are found in parentheses after the main term. A nonessential modifier does not affect selection of the code and is used as guidance. In the section on external causes, the main term and modifiers identify the type of accident or occurrence, vehicle(s) involved, the place of occurrence, and other types of external causes and injuries.

Review Figures 5.1 and 5.2, which are excerpts from the ICD-10-CM Alphabetic Index.

FIGURE 5.1 Excerpts From the ICD-10-CM Alphabetic Index

Acanthamebiasis (with) B60.10
   conjunctiva B60.12   ◄——————— *Indented format Alphabetic Index*
   keratoconjunctivitis B60.13
   meningoencephalitis B60.11
   other specified B60.19

FIGURE 5.2 Excerpts From the ICD-10-CM Alphabetic Index

Hydrarthrosis (*see also* Effusion, joint)
   gonococcal A45.42
   intermittent M12.40
   ankle M12.47-
   elbow M12.42-
   foot joint M12.44-
   hand joint M12.44-
   hip M12.45-
   knee M12.46-
   multiple sites M12.49
   shoulder M12.41-
   specified jpint NEC M12.48
   wrist M12.43-
   of yaws (early) (late) (*see also* subcategory M14.8-) A66.6
   syphilitic A52.77
      congenital A50.55 [M12.80]

Notice that some codes in this category require additional characters. A code in the Alphabetic Index that appears with an ending dash (-) requires additional characters. As with ICD-9-CM, coding should never be selected from the Alphabetic Index. Codes from the Tabular List may have additional instructional notes or character assignment.

Also notice in Figure 5.2 that for the condition *hydrarthrosis*, there is an instructional note *(see also)* referring the user to the condition. In this instance, the condition should be referenced. This instructional note has the same meaning as it did in ICD-9-CM.

Tabular List

The Tabular List (Volume 1) is organized alphanumerically by category and is further subclassified into five-, six-, and seven-character extensions. The indented format of the Tabular List is shown in Figure 5.3.

FIGURE 5.3 Tabular List Indented Format

L71	Rosacea	
	L71.0	Perioral dermatitis ←——————— *Indented format Tabular List*
	L71.1	Rhinophyma
	L71.8	Other rosacea
	L71.9	Rosacea, unspecified

Review the example in Figure 5.3 of the Tabular List indented format.

Notes in ICD-10-CM are similar to those in ICD-9-CM. When a note appears under a three-digit category code, the note applies to all codes within the category. A note that appears beneath a specific code applies only to that particular code.

For example, a patient was diagnosed with hydrarthrosis of the hip. In the Alphabetic Index (Volume 2) of ICD-10-CM, the code category for the hip is M12.45-. The ending dash (-) indicates that additional digits are required, which are referenced in Volume 1 (Tabular List). Figure 5.4 shows an example of the Tabular List.

FIGURE 5.4 Excerpt From ICD-10-CM Tabular List

M12.4	Intermittent hydrarthrosis	
	M12.45	Intermittent hydrarthrosis, hip
		M12.451 Intermittent hydrarthrosis, right hip
		M12.452 Intermittent hydrarthrosis, left hip
		M12.459 Intermittent hydrarthrosis, unspecified hip

In this example, documentation of laterality is important. Code M12.45 has a sixth character extension for right, left, and unspecified hip. Because the scenario does not include identity of the hip, code M12.459 would be the appropriate code selection. As with ICD-9-CM, both the Alphabetic Index and Tabular List must be used.

Chapters

Chapters in ICD-10-CM are similar to those in ICD-9-CM, as they are classified by chapter number and disease. Chapters are further divided into subchapters or blocks containing rubrics, which are three-character codes that represents a single condition or disease, and identifying conditions that are closely related. A summary of the subchapters in each chapter is available in ICD-10-CM and provides an overview of the classification structure. The title of each subchapter describes the subchapter's contents.

Three-Character Categories

The core classification of ICD-10 is the three-character code, and it is the mandatory level of coding for international reporting to the World Health Organization mortality database and for general international comparisons. The four-character subcategories, although not mandatory for reporting at the international level, are recommended for many purposes and form an integral part of the ICD, as do the special tabulation lists. The three-digit classifications are called *blocks* in ICD-10-CM. All three-digit code categories have the same traits. Digits beyond the three alphanumeric codes define a higher level of specificity.

All categories are three characters. Three-character categories define the division between the disease classification and a group of related conditions. The disease categories range from A00 to Z99. These categories may represent a single disease or related conditions. The three-digit category defines the content of the category.

Each character for all categories, subcategories, and codes may be a letter or number. All categories are three characters. The first of every category is an alphabetic character followed by numbers for the second and third characters. A three-character category that has no further subdivision is equivalent to a code. This is similar to instances in ICD-9-CM when a three-digit category cannot be further subdivided to a higher level of specificity.

Review the three-digit categories or blocks in ICD-10-CM by chapter.

Three-Character Categories From ICD-10-CM by Chapter

The three-character categories in ICD-10-CM are outlined below by chapter.

Chapter 1	**Certain infectious and parasitic diseases (A00-B99)**
A00–A09	Intestinal infectious diseases
A15–A19	Tuberculosis
A20–A28	Certain zoonotic bacterial diseases
A30–A49	Other bacterial diseases
A50–A64	Infections with a predominantly sexual mode of transmission

A65–A69	Other spirochetal diseases
A70–A74	Other diseases caused by chlamydiae
A75–A79	Rickettsioses
A80–A89	Viral infections of the central nervous system
A90–A99	Arthropod-borne viral fevers and viral hemorrhagic fevers
B00–B09	Viral infections characterized by skin and mucous membrane lesions
B15–B19	Viral hepatitis
B20–B24	Human immunodeficiency virus [HIV] disease
B25–B34	Other viral diseases
B35–B49	Mycoses
B50–B64	Protozoal diseases
B65–B83	Helminthiases
B85–B89	Pediculosis, acariasis and other infestations
B90–B94	Sequelae of infectious and parasitic diseases
B95–B97	Bacterial, viral and other infectious agents
B99	Other infectious diseases
Chapter 2	**Neoplasms (C00-D49)**
C00–C75	Malignant neoplasms, stated or presumed to be primary, of specified sites, except of lymphoid, hematopoietic and related tissue
C00–C14	Lip, oral cavity and pharynx
C15–C26	Digestive organs
C30–C39	Respiratory and intrathoracic organs
C40–C41	Bone and articular cartilage
C43–C44	Skin
C45–C49	Mesothelial and soft tissue
C50	Breast
C51–C58	Female genital organs
C60–C63	Male genital organs
C64–C68	Urinary tract

C69–C72	Eye, brain and other parts of central nervous system
C73–C75	Thyroid and other endocrine glands
C76–C80	Malignant neoplasms of ill-defined, secondary and unspecified sites
C81–C96	Malignant neoplasms, stated or presumed to be primary, of lymphoid, hematopoietic and related tissue
D00–D09	In situ neoplasms
D10–D36	Benign neoplasms
D37–D48	Neoplasms of uncertain behavior
D49	Neoplasms of unspecified behavior

Chapter 3   **Diseases of the blood and blood-forming organs and certain disorders involving the immune mechanism (D50–D89)**

D50–D53	Nutritional anemias
D55–D59	Hemolytic anemias
D60–D64	Aplastic and other anemias
D65–D69	Coagulation defects, purpura and other hemorrhagic conditions
D70–D78	Other diseases of blood and blood-forming organs
D80–D89	Certain disorders involving the immune mechanism

Chapter 4   **Endocrine, nutritional and metabolic diseases (E00–E90)**

E00–E07	Disorders of thyroid gland
E08–E14	Diabetes mellitus
E15–E16	Other disorders of glucose regulation and pancreatic internal secretion
E20–E36	Disorders of other endocrine glands
E40–E46	Malnutrition
E50–E64	Other nutritional deficiencies
E65–E68	Obesity and other hyperalimentation
E70–E90	Metabolic disorders

Chapter 5   **Mental and behavioral disorders (F01–F99)**

| F01–F09 | Mental disorders due to known physiological conditions |

F10–F19	Mental and behavioral disorders due to psychoactive substance use
F20–F29	Schizophrenia, schizotypal and delusional, and other non-mood psychotic disorders
F30–F39	Mood [affective] disorders
F40–F48	Anxiety, dissociative, stress-related, somatoform and other nonpsychotic mental disorders
F50–F59	Behavioral syndromes associated with physiological disturbances and physical factors
F60–F69	Disorders of adult personality and behavior
F70–F79	Mental retardation
F80–F89	Pervasive and specific developmental disorders
F90–F98	Behavioral and emotional disorders with onset usually occurring in childhood and adolescence
F99	Unspecified mental disorder

Chapter 6 **Diseases of the nervous system (G00–G99)**

G00–G09	Inflammatory diseases of the central nervous system
G10–G13	Systemic atrophies primarily affecting the central nervous system
G20–G26	Extrapyramidal and movement disorders
G30–G32	Other degenerative diseases of the nervous system
G35–G37	Demyelinating diseases of the central nervous system
G40–G47	Episodic and paroxysmal disorders
G50–G59	Nerve, nerve root and plexus disorders
G60–G64	Polyneuropathies and other disorders of the peripheral nervous system
G70–G73	Diseases of myoneural junction and muscle
G80–G83	Cerebral palsy and other paralytic syndromes
G90–G99	Other disorders of the nervous system

Chapter 7 **Disorders of the eye and adnexa (H00-H59)**

H00–H05	Disorders of eyelid, lacrimal system and orbit
H10–H13	Disorders of conjunctiva
H15–H21	Disorders of sclera, cornea, iris and ciliary body

H25–H28	Disorders of lens
H30–H36	Disorders of choroid and retina
H40–H42	Glaucoma
H43–H45	Disorders of vitreous body and globe
H46–H47	Disorders of optic nerve and visual pathways
H49–H52	Disorders of ocular muscles, binocular movement, accommodation and refraction
H53–H54	Visual disturbances and blindness
H55–H59	Other disorders of eye and adnexa

Chapter 8   Diseases of the ear and mastoid process (H60–H95)

H60–H62	Diseases of external ear
H65–H75	Diseases of middle ear and mastoid
H80–H83	Diseases of inner ear
H90–H95	Other disorders of ear

Chapter 9   Diseases of the circulatory system (I00-I99)

I00–I02	Acute rheumatic fever
I05–I09	Chronic rheumatic heart diseases
I10–I15	Hypertensive diseases
I20–I25	Ischemic heart diseases
I26–I28	Pulmonary heart disease and diseases of pulmonary circulation
I30–I52	Other forms of heart disease
I60–I69	Cerebrovascular diseases
I70–I79	Diseases of arteries, arterioles and capillaries
I80–I89	Diseases of veins, lymphatic vessels and lymph nodes, not elsewhere classified
I95–I99	Other and unspecified disorders of the circulatory system

Chapter 10   Diseases of the respiratory system (J00–J99)

J00–J06	Acute upper respiratory infections
J10–J18	Influenza and pneumonia
J20–J22	Other acute lower respiratory infections

J30–J39	Other diseases of upper respiratory tract
J40–J47	Chronic lower respiratory diseases
J60–J70	Lung diseases due to external agents
J80–J84	Other respiratory diseases principally affecting the interstitium
J85–J86	Suppurative and necrotic conditions of the lower respiratory tract
J90–J94	Other diseases of the pleura
J95–J99	Other diseases of the respiratory system

Chapter 11   **Diseases of the digestive system (K00–K94)**

K00–K14	Diseases of oral cavity and salivary glands
K20–K31	Diseases of esophagus, stomach and duodenum
K35–K38	Diseases of appendix
K40–K46	Hernia
K50–K52	Noninfective enteritis and colitis
K55–K63	Other diseases of intestines
K65–K68	Diseases of peritoneum and retroperitoneum
K70–K77	Diseases of liver
K80–K87	Disorders of gallbladder, biliary tract and pancreas
K90–K94	Other diseases of the digestive system

Chapter 12   **Diseases of the skin and subcutaneous tissue (L00–L99)**

L00–L08	Infections of the skin and subcutaneous tissue
L10–L14	Bullous disorders
L20–L30	Dermatitis and eczema
L40–L45	Papulosquamous disorders
L50–L54	Urticaria and erythema
L55–L59	Radiation-related disorders of the skin and subcutaneous tissue
L60–L75	Disorders of skin appendages
L76	Intraoperative and postprocedural complications of dermatologic procedures
L80–L99	Other disorders of the skin and subcutaneous tissue

Chapter 13   **Diseases of the musculoskeletal system and connective tissue (M00–M99)**

M00–M02	Infectious arthropathies
M05–M14	Inflammatory polyarthropathies
M15–M19	Osteoarthritis
M20–M25	Other joint disorders
M26–M27	Dentofacial anomalies [including malocclusion] and other disorders of jaw
M30–M36	Systemic connective tissue disorders
M40–M43	Deforming dorsopathies
M45–M49	Spondylopathies
M50–M54	Other dorsopathies
M60–M63	Disorders of muscles
M65–M67	Disorders of synovium and tendon
M70–M79	Other soft tissue disorders
M80–M85	Disorders of bone density and structure
M86–M90	Other osteopathies
M91–M94	Chondropathies
M95–M99	Other disorders of the musculoskeletal system and connective tissue

Chapter 14   **Diseases of the genitourinary system (N00–N99)**

N00–N08	Glomerular diseases
N10–N16	Renal tubulo-interstitial diseases
N17–N19	Renal failure
N20–N23	Urolithiasis
N25–N29	Other disorders of kidney and ureter
N30–N39	Other diseases of urinary system
N40–N51	Diseases of male genital organs
N60–N64	Disorders of breast
N70–N77	Inflammatory diseases of female pelvic organs
N80–N98	Noninflammatory disorders of female genital tract
N99	Other disorders of genitourinary system

Chapter 15   **Pregnancy, childbirth, and the puerperium (O00–O99)**

O00–O08	Pregnancy with abortive outcome
O09	Supervision of high-risk pregnancy
O10–O16	Edema, proteinuria and hypertensive disorders in pregnancy, childbirth, and the puerperium
O20–O29	Other maternal disorders predominantly related to pregnancy
O30–O48	Maternal care related to the fetus and amniotic cavity and possible delivery problems
O60–O77	Complications of labor and delivery
O80–O82	Encounter for delivery
O85–O92	Complications predominantly related to the puerperium
O93	Sequelae of complication of pregnancy, childbirth, and the puerperium
O94–O99	Other obstetric conditions, not elsewhere classified

Chapter 16   **Certain conditions originating in the perinatal period (P00–P96)**

P00–P04	Newborn affected by maternal factors and by complications of pregnancy, labor and delivery
P05–P08	Disorders related to length of gestation and fetal growth
P10–P15	Birth trauma
P19–P29	Respiratory and cardiovascular disorders specific to the perinatal period
P35–P39	Infections specific to the perinatal period
P50–P61	Hemorrhagic and hematological disorders of newborn
P70–P74	Transitory endocrine and metabolic disorders specific to newborn
P75–P78	Digestive system disorders of newborn
P80–P83	Conditions involving the integument and temperature regulation of newborn
P84	Other problems with newborn
P90–P96	Other disorders originating in the perinatal period

Chapter 17	**Congenital malformations, deformations and chromosomal abnormalities (Q00–Q99)**
Q00–Q07	Congenital malformations of the nervous system
Q10–Q18	Congenital malformations of the eye, ear, face and neck
Q20–Q28	Congenital malformations of the circulatory system
Q30–Q34	Congenital malformations of the respiratory system
Q35–Q37	Cleft lip and cleft palate
Q38–Q45	Other congenital malformations of the digestive system
Q50–Q56	Congenital malformations of genital organs
Q60–Q64	Congenital malformations of the urinary system
Q65–Q79	Congenital malformations and deformations of the musculoskeletal system
Q80–Q89	Other congenital malformations
Q90–Q99	Chromosomal abnormalities, not elsewhere classified
Chapter 18	**Symptoms, signs and abnormal clinical and laboratory findings, not elsewhere classified (R00–R99)**
R00–R09	Symptoms and signs involving the circulatory and respiratory systems
R10–R19	Symptoms and signs involving the digestive system and abdomen
R20–R23	Symptoms and signs involving the skin and subcutaneous tissue
R25–R29	Symptoms and signs involving the nervous and musculoskeletal systems
R30–R39	Symptoms and signs involving the urinary system
R40–R46	Symptoms and signs involving cognition, perception, emotional state and behavior
R47–R49	Symptoms and signs involving speech and voice
R50–R69	General symptoms and signs
R70–R79	Abnormal findings on examination of blood, without diagnosis
R80–R82	Abnormal findings on examination of urine, without diagnosis

R83–R89	Abnormal findings on examination of other body fluids, substances and tissues, without diagnosis
R90–R94	Abnormal findings on diagnostic imaging and in function studies, without diagnosis
R99	Ill-defined and unknown cause of mortality

Chapter 19   **Injury, poisoning and certain other consequences of external cause (S00–T88)**

S00–S09	Injuries to the head
S10–S19	Injuries to the neck
S20–S29	Injuries to the thorax
S30–S39	Injuries to the abdomen, lower back, lumbar spine, pelvis and external genitals
S40–S49	Injuries to the shoulder and upper arm
S50–S59	Injuries to the elbow and forearm
S60–S69	Injuries to the wrist and hand
S70–S79	Injuries to the hip and thigh
S80–S89	Injuries to the knee and lower leg
S90–S99	Injuries to the ankle and foot
T07	Unspecified multiple injuries
T14	Injury of unspecified body region
T15–T19	Effects of foreign body entering through natural orifice
T20–T32	Burns and corrosions
T33–T34	Frostbite
T36–T50	Poisoning by adverse effect of and underdosing of drugs, medicaments and biological substances
T51–T65	Toxic effects of substances chiefly nonmedicinal as to source
T66–T78	Other and unspecified effects of external causes
T79	Certain early complications of trauma
T80–T88	Complications of surgical and medical care, not elsewhere classified

Chapter 20   **External causes of morbidity (V01–Y98)**

V00–X58	Accidents

V00–V99	Transport accidents
V00–V09	Pedestrian injured in transport accident
V10–V19	Pedal cyclist injured in transport accident
V20–V29	Motorcycle rider injured in transport accident
V30–V39	Occupant of three-wheeled motor vehicle injured in transport accident
V40–V49	Car occupant injured in transport accident
V50–V59	Occupant of pick-up truck or van injured in transport accident
V60–V69	Occupant of heavy transport vehicle injured in transport accident
V70–V79	Bus occupant injured in transport accident
V80–V89	Other land transport accidents
V90–V94	Water transport accidents
V95–V97	Air and space transport accidents
V98–V99	Other and unspecified transport accidents
W00–X58	Other external causes of accidental injury
W00–W19	Falls
W20–W49	Exposure to inanimate mechanical forces
W50–W64	Exposure to animate mechanical forces
W65–W74	Accidental drowning and submersion
W85–W99	Exposure to electric current, radiation and extreme ambient air temperature and pressure
X00–X09	Exposure to smoke, fire and flames
X10–X19	Contact with heat and hot substances
X30–X39	Exposure to forces of nature
X52, X58	Accidental exposure to other specified factors
X71–X83	Intentional self-harm
X92–Y08	Assault
Y21–Y33	Event of undetermined intent
Y35–Y38	Legal intervention, operations of war, military operations and terrorism

Y62–Y84	Complications of medical and surgical care
Y62–Y69	Misadventures to patients during surgical and medical care
Y70–Y82	Medical devices associated with adverse incidents in diagnostic and therapeutic use
Y83–Y84	Surgical and other medical procedures as the cause of abnormal reaction of the patient, or of later complication, without mention of misadventure at the time of the procedure
Y90–Y98	Supplementary factors related to causes of morbidity classified elsewhere
Chapter 21	**Factors influencing health status and contact with health services (Z00–Z99)**
Z00–Z13	Persons encountering health services for examination and investigation
Z14–Z15	Genetic carrier and genetic susceptibility to disease
Z16	Infection with drug-resistant microorganisms
Z20–Z28	Persons with potential health hazards related to communicable diseases
Z30–Z39	Persons encountering health services in circumstances related to reproduction
Z40–Z53	Persons encountering health services for specific procedures and health care
Z55–Z65	Persons with potential health hazards related to socioeconomic and psychosocial circumstances
Z66	Do not resuscitate (DNR) status
Z67	Blood type
Z69–Z76	Persons encountering health services in other circumstances
Z79–Z99	Persons with potential health hazards related to family and personal history and certain conditions influencing health status

Review the example of three-digit categories in ICD-10-CM Chapter 3. Figure 5.5 illustrates the format of three-digit categories or blocks.

FIGURE 5.5 Three-Digit Categories

Diseases of the blood and blood-forming organs and certain disorders involving the immune mechanism (D50-D89)

D50–D53	Nutritional anemias
D55–D59	Hemolytic anemias
D60–D64	Aplastic and other anemias and other bone marrow failure syndromes
D65–D69	Coagulation defects, purpura and other hemorrhagic conditions
D70–D77	Other disorders of blood and blood-forming organs
D78	Intraoperative and postprocedural complications of spleen
D80–D89	Certain disorders involving the immune mechanism

Review the three-digit categories within the chapter. Figure 5.6 illustrates the format of three-digit categories within the chapter blocks.

FIGURE 5.6 Three-Digit Categories

D50	Iron deficiency anemia
D51	Vitamin B_{12} deficiency anemia
D52	Folate deficiency anemia
D53	Other nutritional anemias

Subcategories are either four or five characters with codes of either four, five, or six characters. Each level after the category is a subcategory and can be further defined to the fourth, fifth, or sixth level of specificity.

Four-Character Subclassification

Four-digit subcategories define the site, etiology, manifestation, or state of the disease or condition. The four-digit subcategory includes the three-digit category plus a decimal point with an additional digit to further identify the condition to the highest level of specificity.

Below are examples of the various code levels:

A17.8	Other tuberculosis of nervous system
K13.5	Other submucous fibrosis
O75.5	Delayed delivery after artificial rupture of membranes
S12.030	Displaced posterior arch fracture of first cervical vertebra

Below some examples of four-digit codes applied to various diseases.

Example: Diseases of the Breast

N60   Benign mammary dysplasia

> Excludes1: Disorders of breast associated with childbirth
> (O91-O92)

N60.1   Diffuse cystic mastopathy

N60.2   Fibroadenosis of breast

N60.3   Fibrosclerosis of breast

N60.4   Mammary duct ectasia

N60.8   Other benign mammary dysplasias

N60.9   Unspecified benign mammary dysplasia

Notice that there is an *Excludes1* note indicating that any disorder of the breast associated with childbirth is never coded in this category. An *Excludes1* note indicates that the code is excluded and should never be used at the same time as the code above the *Excludes1* note. An *Excludes1* note is for use when two conditions cannot occur together, such as a congenital form versus an acquired form of the same condition.

Example: Histoplasmosis

B39   Histoplasmosis

> Code first associated AIDS (B20)

> Use additional code for any associated manifestations, such as:
> endocarditis (I39)
> meningitis (G02)
> pericarditis (I32)
> retinitis (H32)

B39.0   Acute pulmonary histoplasmosis capsulati

B39.1   Chronic pulmonary histoplasmosis capsulati

B39.2   Pulmonary histoplasmosis capsulati, unspecified

B39.3   Disseminated histoplasmosis capsulati
            Generalized histoplasmosis capsulati

B39.4   Histoplasmosis capsulati, unspecified
            American histoplasmosis

B39.5   Histoplasmosis duboisii
            African histoplasmosis

B39.9   Histoplasmosis, unspecified

In this example, the instructional note indicates to first code associated AIDS from category B20 and to use an additional code for associated manifestations. These instructional notes should be followed in ICD-10-CM, if the condition(s) is/are supported in the medical record.

Five-Character and Six-Character Subclassifications

In ICD-9-CM, the fifth digit identifies the most precise level of specificity. In ICD-10-CM, a fifth or sixth character subclassification represents the most accurate level of specificity. This addition may identify more specificity regarding the patient's condition or diagnosis.

Example: Tympanosclerosis

A patient visited an otologist with a complaint of right ear pain that had become chronic. After examination of the patient, the physician diagnosed tympanosclerosis of the right ear with chronic mastoiditis. The encounter is reported as follows: the principal/first listed diagnosis is H74.01 (Tympanosclerosis, right ear), and the secondary diagnosis is H70.11 (Chronic mastoiditis, right ear).

The codes for tympanosclerosis are as follows:

H74   Other disorders of middle ear and mastoid

      Excludes2: Mastoiditis (H70.-)

    H74.0   Tympanosclerosis
       H74.01 Tympanosclerosis, right ear
       H74.02 Tympanosclerosis, left ear
       H74.03 Tympanosclerosis, bilateral
       H74.09 Tympanosclerosis, unspecified ear

Also take note that there is an *Excludes2* notation indicating that the condition excluded is not part of the condition it is excluded from, but a patient may have both conditions at the same time. When an *Excludes2* note appears under a code, it is acceptable to use both the code and the excluded code together. Also, when coding is done with subcategory H74-, documentation of laterality is important in the code selection, so the unspecified ear code is not used.

Example: Hypertensive Heart Disease

The codes for hypertensive heart disease are as follows:

I11   Hypertensive heart disease

      Includes: any condition in I51.4-I51.9 due to hypertension

    I11.0   Hypertensive heart disease with heart failure
       Hypertensive heart failure

Use additional code to identify type of heart failure (I50.-)

  I11.9 Hypertensive heart disease without heart failure
       Hypertensive heart disease NOS

Notice in this example that there is a note to use an additional code to identify the type of heart failure, with I11.0 for the hypertensive heart disease with heart failure using subcategory I50-.

Example: Pain in Upper Extremity

A writer who spends hours typing at the computer was experiencing constant pain in her right arm. In ICD-10-CM, the encounter is reported using a six-character subclassification. The codes are as follows:

 M79.6 Pain in limb, hand, foot, fingers and toes

    Excludes2: Pain in joint (M25.5-)

  M79.60 Pain in limb, unspecified
    M79.601 Pain in right arm
       Pain in right upper limb NOS
    M79.602 Pain in left arm
       Pain in left upper limb NOS
    M79.603 Pain in arm, unspecified
       Pain in upper limb NOS

In this example, the correct code to report is M79.601 for pain in the right arm. Notice the *Excludes2* note is applicable to this category to identify pain in the joint if documented. Because joint pain is not documented in the example, the joint pain would not be reported.

Seven-Character Subclassification

Chapter 19 of ICD-10-CM contains the codes for injuries and poisoning and other consequences of external causes. This chapter is divided into two sections, the *S* codes and *T* codes. The S codes are the traumatic injury codes. The T codes are for burns and corrosions, poisonings and toxic effects and underdosing, complications of medical care, and other such consequences of external causes. These codes are typically six and seven characters, with some codes requiring character extensions. Character extensions are defined at the category level of ICD-10-CM in the Tabular List.

Example: Laceration to Arm

A 45-year-old male was rushed to an emergency department after accidentally slashing his right arm with a sharp knife while attempting to clean fish he caught while deep-sea fishing in the Caribbean. The diagnosis reported by the emergency department physician was a laceration of the ulnar artery at the forearm level, right arm. The codes are as follows:

S55   Injury of blood vessels at forearm level
Code also any associated open wound (S51.-)
Excludes2: injury of blood vessels at wrist and hand level (S65.-)
injury of brachial vessels (S45.1-S45.2)

The following seven-character extensions are to be added to each code for category S55:

A   initial encounter
D   subsequent encounter
S   sequela

S55.0   Injury of ulnar artery at forearm level
S55.00   Unspecified injury of ulnar artery at forearm level
S55.001   Unspecified injury of ulnar artery at forearm level, right arm
S55.002   Unspecified injury of ulnar artery at forearm level, left arm
S55.009   Unspecified injury of ulnar artery at forearm level, unspecified arm

S55.01   Laceration of ulnar artery at forearm level
S55.011   Laceration of ulnar artery at forearm level, right arm
S55.012   Laceration of ulnar artery at forearm level, left arm
S55.019   Laceration of ulnar artery at forearm level, unspecified arm

S55.09   Other specified injury of ulnar artery at forearm level
S55.091   Other specified injury of ulnar artery at forearm level, right arm
S55.092   Other specified injury of ulnar artery at forearm level, left arm
S55.099   Other specified injury of ulnar artery

The correct code selection for this example would be S55.011a (Laceration of ulnar artery at the right forearm, initial encounter). The seventh character extension is required for coding in this category. The instructional notes also instruct the coder to report the open wound. Because the documentation indicated the laceration, the open wound would also be reported. Guidance also directs the coder to report as a seven-character extension whether the laceration is initial (A), subsequent (D), or a sequela (S). The principal or first listed diagnosis would be S55.011a (Laceration of ulnar artery at the right forearm, initial encounter), and the secondary diagnosis would be S51.811a (Laceration without foreign body of right forearm, initial encounter).

Notice that the diagnosis code S55.001 (six-digit subclassification) details the type of injury, site of injury, and what side of the body, if affected. Also notice that a seventh digit is required to indicate that the condition is the first encounter for the treatment or injury (A), a complication or condition arising as a result of the injury (S), or a subsequent encounter (D), which may be used for as long as the patient is receiving treatment for an injury.

Also take note that there is an *Excludes2* notation, which indicates that the condition excluded is not part of the condition it is excluded from, but a patient may have both conditions at the same time. When an *Excludes2* note appears under a code, it is acceptable to use both the code and the excluded code together.

Extensions

ICD-10-CM also uses a "dummy placeholder," which is always the letter *x*. The dummy placeholder is used as a fifth character placeholder in certain six-character codes to allow for further expansion. Some examples of where dummy placeholders are used can be found in categories T36-T50 (poisoning codes) and categories T51-T65 (toxic effect codes), as illustrated in Figure 5.7.

Review in Figure 5.7 the subcategory, poisoning by adverse effect of and underdosing of anticoagulant antagonists, vitamin K, and other coagulants (T45.7).

FIGURE 5.7 Excerpt From ICD-10-CM Tabular List With x Dummy Placeholders

T45.7   Poisoning by, adverse effect of, and underdosing of anticoagulant antagonists, vitamin K, and other coagulants

 T45.7x   Poisoning by, adverse effect of, and underdosing of anticoagulant antagonists, vitamin K, and other coagulants

 Excludes1: Vitamin K deficiency (E56.1)

  T45.7x1   Poisoning by anticoagulant antagonists, vitamin K, and other coagulants, accidental (unintentional)
   Poisoning by anticoagulant antagonists, vitamin K, and other coagulants NOS

  T45.7x2   Poisoning by anticoagulant antagonists, vitamin K, and other coagulants, intentional self-harm

  T45.7x3   Poisoning by anticoagulant antagonists, vitamin K, and other coagulants, assault

  T45.7x4   Poisoning by anticoagulant antagonists, vitamin K, and other coagulants, undetermined

  T45.7x5   Adverse effect of anticoagulant antagonists, vitamin K, and other coagulants

  T45.7x6   Underdosing of anticoagulant antagonist, vitamin K, and other coagulants

---

The fifth character in T45.7 in Figure 5.6 identifies a dummy placeholder. The dummy placeholder is identified with an "x". The fifth character placeholder is to allow for future expansion without disturbing the six-character structure. The fifth-character placeholder indicates the intent as:

- unintentional (accident);
- intentional self-harm;
- assault;
- undetermined;
- adverse effect; or
- underdosing.

For example, a patient experienced an adverse effect of an antineoplastic and immunosuppressive drug. The initial encounter was coded as T45.1x5a (Adverse effect of antineoplastic and immunosuppressive drugs, initial encounter). The seventh character, *a*, identifies the visit as the initial encounter.

Review the Figure 5.8 example of the T45 category for poisoning by adverse effect of an underdosing of primary systemic and hematological agents, not elsewhere classified.

FIGURE 5.8 Excerpt From ICD-10-CM Tabular List Category T45

T45   Poisoning by, adverse effect of, and underdosing of primarily systemic and hematological agents, not elsewhere classified

The appropriate seventh character is to be added to each code from category T45

    A   initial encounter
    D   subsequent encounter
    S   sequela

  T45.1 Poisoning by, adverse effect of, and underdosing of antineoplastic and immunosuppressive drugs

        Excludes1: Poisoning by, adverse effect of, and underdosing of tamoxifen (T38.6)

      T45.1x Poisoning by, adverse effect of and underdosing of antineoplastic and immunosuppressive drugs

          T45.1x1 Poisoning by antineoplastic and immunosuppressive drugs, accidental (unintentional)

                Poisoning by antineoplastic and immunosuppressive drugs NOS

          T45.1x2 Poisoning by antineoplastic and immunosuppressive drugs, intentional self-harm

          T45.1x3 Poisoning by antineoplastic and immunosuppressive drugs, assault

          T45.1x4 Poisoning by antineoplastic and immunosuppressive drugs, undetermined

          T45.1x5 Adverse effect of antineoplastic and immunosuppressive drugs

          T45.1x6 Underdosing of antineoplastic and immunosuppressive drugs

Conventions Used in ICD-10-CM

Many of the conventions in ICD-9-CM will be used in ICD-10-CM, which will help make the conversion easier.

Brackets

Brackets are used in the Tabular List to enclose synonyms, alternative wording, or explanatory phrases. Brackets are used in the Alphabetic Index to identify manifestation codes (*see Code First/Use additional code convention*).

Below is an example of the use of brackets:

D68.2 Hereditary deficiency of other clotting factors
AC globulin deficiency
Congenital afibrinogenemia deficiency of factor I [fibrinogen]
Deficiency of factor II [prothrombin]
Deficiency of factor V [labile]
Deficiency of factor VII [stable]
Deficiency of factor X [Stuart-Prower]
Deficiency of factor XII [Hageman]
Deficiency of factor XIII [ibrin stabilizing]
Dysfibrinogenemia (congenital)
Proaccelerin deficiency

In this example, the brackets are used to further define the terminology of the code.

Parentheses

Parentheses are used in both the Index and Tabular List to enclose supplementary words that may be present or absent in the statement of a disease or procedure without affecting the code number to which it is assigned. The terms within the parentheses are referred to as *nonessential modifiers*. An example of the use of parentheses in the Alphabetic Index would be, "Deuteranopia (complete) (incomplete) H53.53." An example of the use of parentheses in the Tabular List is shown below:

E76.29 Other mucopolysaccharidoses
Beta-glucuronidase deficiency
Maroteaux-Lamy (mild) (severe) syndrome
Mucopolysaccharidosis, types VI, VII

In this case, the parentheses identify supplementary words (*mild* and *severe*) that are not required in documentation to report the code.

Colon

A colon is used in the Tabular List after an incomplete term that needs one or more of the modifiers following the colon to make it assignable to a given category.

And

When the term *and* is used in a narrative statement, it represents and/or when a code is being selected.

See

The instruction *see* acts as a cross-reference and directs the user to look elsewhere. This instruction is often found when the term or condition may not be the appropriate term. This is a mandatory instruction and must be followed for proper code selection (eg, "Ankylostoma – **See** ancylostoma, ancylostomiasis; **see** ancylostomiasis" or "Ankylurethria – **See** stricture, urethra").

See also

See also is a reference instructional note to refer to a specific category, subcategory, or subclassification before making a code selection if the diagnosis listed cannot be found under a term. Some examples are below:

> Amentia – ***See also*** retardation, mental
> Meynert's (nonalcoholic) F04
> Annular – ***See also*** condition

Not Elsewhere Classified

Not elsewhere classified (NEC) codes titled *Other* or *Other specified* in the Tabular List (usually a code with a fourth or sixth character 8 or Z and fifth character 9) are for use when the information in the medical record provides detail for which a specific code does not exist. The abbreviation *NEC* represents *other specified* in ICD-10-CM. An Alphabetic Index entry that states *NEC* directs the coder to an *other specified* code in the Tabular List (see inclusion terms).

Below is an example from the Alphabetic Index:

> Abruptio placentae O45.9-
> – with
>> – afibrinogenemia O45.01
>> – coagulation defect O45.00
>> – specified **NEC** O45.09
>> – disseminated intravascular coagulation O45.02
>> – hypofibrinogenemia O45.01
>> – specified **NEC** O45.8x

Not Otherwise Specified "Unspecified" Codes

Codes in the Tabular List with *unspecified* in the title (usually a code with a fourth or sixth character 9 and fifth character 0) are for use when the information in the medical record is insufficient to assign a more specific code.

The abbreviation *NOS* in the Tabular List is the equivalent of unspecified. An example is shown below:

F10.988   Alcohol use, **unspecified** with other alcohol-induced disorder

K31.1   Adult hypertrophic pyloric stenosis
     Pyloric stenosis NOS

Includes

The word *includes* appears immediately under certain categories to further define, or give examples of, the content of the category. An example is shown below:

> **Certain disorders involving the immune mechanism (D80–D89)**
> **Includes:** defects in the complement system, ◄—— *Applies to code*
>   immunodeficiency disorders, except human immunodefi-
>   ciency virus [HIV] disease, sarcoidosis
> Excludes1: autoimmune disease (systemic) NOS (M35.9)

Excludes Notes

The ICD-10-CM has two types of *excludes* notes. Each note has a different definition for use, but they are both similar in that they indicate that codes excluded from each other are independent of each other. An example is below:

S51.05   Open bite of elbow
     Bite of elbow NOS
       Excludes: Superficial bite of elbow (S50.36, S50.37) ◄— *Applies to code*

An *Excludes1* note indicates that the code is excluded and should never be used at the same time as the code above the *Excludes1* note. An *Excludes1* note is for use when two conditions cannot occur together, such as a congenital form versus an acquired form of the same condition. An example is shown below:

I72.0   Aneurysm of carotid artery (common) (external) (internal, extracranial portion)
       Excludes1: Aneurysm of internal carotid artery, intracranial portion (I67.1)
           Aneurysm of internal carotid artery NOS (I67.1)

An *Excludes2* notation indicates that the condition excluded is not part of the condition it is excluded from, but a patient may have both conditions at the same time. When an *Excludes2* note appears under a code, it is acceptable to use both the code and the excluded code together. An example is shown below:

J04.1   Acute tracheitis
     Acute viral tracheitis
     Catarrhal tracheitis (acute)
     Tracheitis (acute) NOS
       Excludes2: Chronic tracheitis (J42)

Code First/Use Additional Code

A *code first/use additional code* notes etiology/manifestation paired codes. Certain conditions have both an underlying etiology and multiple body system manifestations because of the underlying etiology. For such conditions, ICD-10-CM has a coding convention that requires that the underlying condition be sequenced first, followed by the manifestation. Wherever such a combination exists, there is a *use additional code* note at the etiology code and a *code first* note at the manifestation code. These instructional notes indicate the proper sequencing order of the codes, etiology followed by manifestation. In most cases, the manifestation codes will have *in diseases classified elsewhere* in the code title. Codes with this title are a component of the etiology/manifestation convention. The code title indicates that it is a manifestation code. *In diseases classified elsewhere* codes are never permitted to be used as first listed or principle diagnosis codes. They must be used in conjunction with an underlying condition code, and they must be listed following the underlying condition. An example is shown below:

> **H42** Glaucoma in diseases classified elsewhere
> **Code first** underlying disease, such as: ⟵———— *Applies to code*
> Amyloidosis (E85.-)
> Aniridia (Q13.1)
> Lowe's syndrome (E72.03)
> Reiger's anomaly (Q13.81)
> Specified Metabolic Disorders (E70-E90)

Code Also

A *code also* note instructs that two codes may be required to fully describe a condition, but the sequencing of the two codes is discretionary, depending on the severity of the conditions and the reason for the encounter. An example is shown below:

> **J10.1** Influenza due to other influenza virus with respiratory manifestations
> Acute influenzal upper respiratory infection due to other
> influenza virus
> Influenza NOS
> Influenzal laryngitis due to other influenza virus
> Influenzal pharyngitis due to other influenza virus
> Influenzal pleural effusion due to other influenza virus
> **Code also** any associated pneumonia (J12-J18)

With/Without Note

When *with* and *without* are the two options for the final character of a set of codes, the default is always *without*. For five-character codes, 0 as the fifth position character represents *without*, and 1 represents *with*. For six-character codes, the sixth position character 1 represents *with*, and 9 represents *without*. An example of the use of *with* is, "G40.501, Special epileptic syndromes, not intractable, **with** status epilepticus." An example of the use of *without* is, "G40.519, Special epileptic syndromes, intractable, **without** status epilepticus."

After Table 5.2 is reviewed, it will become evident that many of the symbols, terminology, and conventions of ICD-9-D-CM will carry over to ICD-10-CM.

Tabular List Convention Comparison

Review the comparison between ICD-9-CM and ICD-10-CM conventions in Table 5.2. The conventions in ICD-10-CM are similar to those in ICD-9-CM, as shown in Table 5.2.

TABLE 5.2 **Convention Comparison Between ICD-9-CM and ICD-10-CM**		
Convention	**ICD-9-CM**	**ICD-10-CM**
Notes	They further define terms, clarify information, or list choices for additional digits.	They further define terms, clarify information, or list choices for additional digits. *With/without* notes are the two options for the final character of a set of codes; the default is *without*. For five-character codes, 0 as the fifth position character represents *without*, and 1 represents *with*. For six-character codes, the sixth position character 1 represents with, and 9 represents *without*.
Includes	These are notes that further define or provide examples and can apply to the chapter, section, or category. The notes at the beginning of a chapter apply to the entire chapter, the notes at the beginning of the section apply to that entire section, and the notes at the beginning of the category apply to the entire category.	Same as ICD-9-CM

TABLE 5.2 Convention Comparison Between ICD-9-CM and ICD-10-CM *(continued)*

Convention	ICD-9-CM	ICD-10-CM
Not otherwise specified	*Not otherwise specified* (NOS) is the equivalent of *unspecified*. It is used when the information at hand does not permit a more specific code assignment. The coder should ask the physician for more specific information, if available, so that the proper code assignment can be made.	Same as ICD-9-CM
Excludes	These are notes that indicate terms that are to be coded elsewhere. *Excludes notes* can be located at the beginning of a chapter or section or below a category or subcategory and are always italicized. *Excludes notes* can be used for three reasons: **1** The condition may have to be coded elsewhere. **2** The code cannot be assigned if the associated condition is present. **3** Additional code(s) may be required to fully explain the condition.	Same as ICD-9-CM
Code first underlying disease	*Code first underlying disease* is used in those categories not intended as the primary diagnosis. In such cases, the code, title, and instructions appear in italics. The note requires that the underlying cause (etiology) be sequenced first.	Same as ICD-9-CM
Use additional code	This note appears in categories in which further information must be added (by using an additional code) to give a more complete picture of the diagnosis or procedure.	Same as ICD-9-CM

TABLE 5.2 Convention Comparison Between ICD-9-CM and ICD-10-CM *(continued)*

Convention	ICD-9-CM	ICD-10-CM
: Colon	A colon is used after an incomplete term that needs one or more of the modifiers that follow to make it assignable to a given category.	Same as ICD-9-CM
[ ] Brackets	Brackets enclose synonyms, alternate wording, or explanatory phrases.	Same as ICD-9-CM
( ) Parentheses	Parentheses enclose supplementary words that may be present or absent in the statement of a disease or procedure, without affecting the code number to which it is assigned.	Same as ICD-9-CM
{ } Braces	Braces enclose a series of terms, each of which is modified by the statement appearing at the right of the brace.	No braces are used in ICD-10-CM.
, Comma	Words following a comma are essential modifiers. The term in the inclusion note must be present in the diagnostic statement to qualify the code.	Same as ICD-9-CM
§ Section mark	A section mark precedes a code to denote a footnote at the bottom of the page. The footnote applies to all codes in the subclassification.	Same as ICD-9-CM
And	The convention *and* is not used in ICD-9-CM.	When the term *and* is used in a narrative statement, it represents and/or.

Convention	ICD-9-CM	ICD-10-CM
TABLE 5.2 **Convention Comparison Between ICD-9-CM and ICD-10-CM** *(continued)*		
Excludes1	*Excludes* conventions are not used in ICD-9-CM.	*Excludes1* indicates that the code excluded should never be used at the same time as the code above the *Excludes1* note. An *Excludes1* is used when two conditions cannot occur together, such as a congenital form versus an acquired form of the same condition.
Excludes 2	*Excludes* conventions are not used in ICD-9-CM.	An *Excludes2* note represents *not included here.* An *Excludes2* note indicates that the condition excluded is not part of the condition represented by the code, but a patient may have both conditions at the same time. When an *Excludes2* note appears under a code, it is acceptable to use both the code and the excluded code together.

Laterality

For bilateral sites, the final character of the codes in ICD-10-CM indicates laterality. The right side is always character 1, and the left side is character 2. When a bilateral code is applicable, the bilateral character is always 3. An unspecified side code is also provided, should the side not be identified in the medical record. The unspecified side is either a character 0 or 9, depending on whether it is a fifth or sixth character. Laterality is found in many chapters of ICD-10-CM.

For example, a patient sees a physician for follow-up for an abscess of a bursa on the left wrist. The applicable codes are as follows:

> M71.03   Abscess of bursa, wrist
> M71.031   Abscess of bursa, right wrist
> M71.032   Abscess of bursa, left wrist
> M71.039   Abscess of bursa, unspecified wrist

The correct code selection is M71.032 for this patient encounter, because the left wrist is involved.

Summary

The structure and format of ICD-10-CM includes an alphanumeric, indented format with the addition of six-character and seven-character extensions. Another difference between ICD-9-CM and ICD-10-CM is the use of dummy placeholders for further expansion of the fifth character in some of the code categories. Certain categories also have seven-character extensions unique to the category, used for further definition of the code. Conventions used in ICD-10-CM are similar to those used in ICD-9-CM, except the addition of the *Excludes1* and *Excludes2* conventions not used in ICD-9-CM.

Resources

ICD-10-CM *Official Guidelines for Coding and Reporting, 2009.* Available online at the National Center for Health Statistics at ftp://ftp.cdc.gov/pub/ Health_Statistics/NCHS/Publications/ICD10CM/2009/.

National Center for Health Statistics. *ICD-10-CM Alphabetic Index.* Available online at ftp://ftp.cdc.gov/pub/Health_Statistics/NCHS/Publications/ ICD10CM/2009/.

National Center for Health Statistics. *ICD-10-CM Tabular List.* Available online at ftp://ftp.cdc.gov/pub/Health_Statistics/NCHS/Publications/ ICD10CM/2009/.

Grider, Deborah. *Principles of ICD-9-CM.* 2007. 4th Edition. Chicago: AMA Press.

End-of-Chapter Questions

1   The Alphabetic Index in ICD-10-CM is divided into what two parts?

_____ and _____

2   Chapters are further divided into _____.

3   ICD-10-CM uses dummy placeholders defined by the letter _____.

4   The *Excludes1* convention indicates _____.

5   The *Excludes2* convention indicates _____.

CHAPTER 6

ICD-10-CM: General and Chapter-Specific Guidelines for Chapters 1 to 6

OBJECTIVES

- Review *ICD-10-CM Official Guidelines for Coding and Reporting, 2009*
- Understand chapter-specific guidelines and their use
- Review examples of the International Classification of Diseases, Tenth Revision, Clinical Modification (ICD-10-CM) codes relative to the guidelines
- Review comparisons between the International Classification of Diseases, Ninth Revision, Clinical Modification (ICD-9-CM) and ICD-10-CM

Introduction

This chapter will cover the general coding guidelines that pertain to all chapters of ICD-10-CM. It is important to understand the chapter guidelines prior to implementation, which will assist users with documentation-related issues. It is also important to understand the *ICD-10-CM Official Guidelines for Coding and Reporting, 2009.*

Also covered are the chapter-specific guidelines for the following:
- Chapter 1 – Infectious and parasitic diseases
- Chapter 2 – Neoplasms
- Chapter 3 – Diseases of the blood and blood-forming organs and certain disorders involving immune mechanism
- Chapter 4 – Endocrine, nutritional and metabolic diseases
- Chapter 5 – Mental and behavioral disorders
- Chapter 6 – Diseases of the nervous system.

The ICD-10-CM Official Guidelines were published in January 2009. The Alphabetic Index and Tabular List were also updated in January 2009. The guidelines are organized into several sections:
- Section 1 – ICD-10-CM conventions
- Section 2 – General coding guidelines
- Section 3 – Chapter-specific guidelines.

The ICD-10-CM official guidelines are a set of rules that have been developed to accompany and complement the official conventions and instructions provided within ICD-10-CM itself. These guidelines are based on the coding and sequencing instructions in Volumes I and II of ICD-10-CM and provide additional instruction.

Adherence to ICD-10-CM guidelines when assigning ICD-10-CM diagnosis codes is required under the Health Insurance Portability and Accountability Act. The diagnosis codes (Volumes 1-2) have been adopted under the Act for all health care settings. The ICD-10-CM guidelines have been developed to assist both the health care provider and coder in identifying diagnoses that are to be reported. The official guidelines emphasize that complete and consistent documentation in the medical record is vitally important and that without it, accurate coding cannot be achieved. One common term used throughout the official guidelines is *provider*, which means a physician or any qualified health care practitioner who is legally accountable for establishing the patient's diagnosis. Another common term in the official guidelines is *encounter*, which means all settings, including hospital admissions.

Chapter-specific guidelines are sequenced the same as they appear in the Tabular List. To understand rules and instructions in ICD-10-CM, it is necessary to review all sections of the guidelines. This chapter will cover Sections 2 and 3. The Section 1 conventions were covered in Chapter 5. Also covered in this chapter will be a comparison between ICD-9-CM and ICD-10-CM codes.

The ICD-10-CM guidelines are similar in some respects to those of ICD-9-CM but are specific to this coding classification.

General Coding Guidelines

Diagnoses reported in the medical record remain the responsibility of the rendering provider. A joint effort between the provider and the coder is essential in reporting accurate documentation and code selection. Guidelines in ICD-10-CM were developed to assist the provider and coder in assigning the appropriate diagnosis codes.

As with ICD-9-CM, when a code is being given in ICD-10-CM, the term should be located in the Alphabetic Index, then verified in the Tabular List. The user must read all instructional notes in both the Alphabetic Index and Tabular List and verify that the documentation in the medical record supports the code assigned. Keep in mind that the Alphabetic Index does not always provide the complete code. Selection of a diagnosis code in ICD-10-CM includes laterality and further extensions, which are found in the Tabular List. A dash (-) at the end of an Alphabetic Index entry indicates that additional characters are required. Even if a dash is not included in the Alphabetic Index, the user should never code from this volume and always reference the Tabular List for the final code selection.

Signs and Symptoms

As with ICD-9-CM, sign and symptom codes should not be reported with a confirmed diagnosis if the symptom is integral to the diagnosis. For example, if the patient is experiencing ear pain, and the diagnosis is otitis media, the ear pain would be integral to the otitis media and not reported. A symptom code is used with a confirmed diagnosis only when the symptom is not associated with the confirmed diagnosis.

Consider this example of the code differences between ICD-9-CM and ICD-10-CM: A patient was diagnosed with epigastric pain. The physician referred the patient to a gastroenterologist to rule out an ulcer. In ICD-9-CM, the code to report would be 789.06 (Abdominal pain, epigastric). In ICD-10-CM, the code is R10.13 (Epigastric pain).

Sign and symptom codes are generally located in Chapter 18 of ICD-10-CM but may also be located in the body system chapters. Sign and symptom codes are not to be used when a definitive diagnosis related to the signs and symptoms can be reported.

Acute, Subacute, and Chronic Conditions

The guidelines for ICD-10-CM are the same as those for ICD-9-CM regarding encounters with patients with an acute, subacute, and/or a chronic condition.

The ICD-10-CM guidelines state, "When a condition is documented as both acute, subacute, and chronic and separate codes exist in the Indentation level, both are coded with the acute (subacute) sequenced first followed by the code for the chronic condition."

For example, a patient was diagnosed with acute maxillary sinusitis that is chronic. The physician examined the patient and prescribed medication for the condition and asked the patient to return for follow-up in one week. In ICD-10-CM, both codes for the acute and chronic condition are reported. Review code J01 for acute sinusitis in ICD-10-CM and J32 for chronic sinusitis in Figures 6.1 and 6.2.

> **GUIDELINE TIP**
>
> A sign or symptom code is to be used only if no definitive diagnosis is established at the time the patient encounter is coded. When the diagnosis is confirmed prior to coding of the encounter, the confirmed diagnosis is reported.

FIGURE 6.1 Excerpt From ICD-10-CM Tabular List

J01   Acute sinusitis

      Includes: acute abscess of sinus

              acute empyema of sinus

              acute infection of sinus

              acute inflammation of sinus

              acute suppuration of sinus

      Use additional code (B95-B97) to identify infectious agent.

      Excludes1: sinusitis NOS (J32.9)

      Excludes2: chronic sinusitis (J32.0-J32.8)

    J01.0   Acute maxillary sinusitis

        Acute antritis

        J01.00   Acute maxillary sinusitis, unspecified

        J01.01   Acute recurrent maxillary sinusitis

FIGURE 6.2 **Excerpt From ICD-10-CM Tabular List**

J32   Chronic sinusitis
Includes: sinus abscess
        sinus empyema
        sinus infection
        sinus suppuration
Use additional code to identify:
        exposure to environmental tobacco smoke (Z72.22)
        exposure to tobacco smoke in the perinatal period (P96.81)
        history of tobacco use (Z87.891)
        infectious agent (B95-B97)
        occupational exposure to environmental tobacco smoke (Z57.31)
        tobacco dependence (F17.-)
        tobacco use (Z72.0)
Excludes2: acute sinusitis (J01.-)
      J32.0   Chronic maxillary sinusitis
          Antritis (chronic)
          Maxillary sinusitis NOS

The correct diagnosis coding and reporting is:

- J01.00   Acute maxillary sinusitis, unspecified
- J32.0   Chronic maxillary sinusitis.

There is an *Excludes2* note, which indicates that conditions listed with *Excludes2* are not considered inclusive to a code, but may be coexistent, and if present, should also be coded. If acute (subacute) or chronic is documented in the medical record, it would be appropriate, on the basis of ICD-10-CM guidelines, to report both codes.

Combination Coding

Combination codes are a single code to classify two diagnoses and include a diagnosis with an associated sign/symptom or a complication. Combination codes are identified by subordinate term entries in the Alphabetic Index and by the *includes* and *excludes* notes in the Tabular List.

There are many combination codes that include both the etiology and an acute manifestation, in which case the single combination code is assigned as the principal/first listed diagnosis, and no sequencing decision is necessary. Assign only the combination code when that code fully identifies the diagnostic conditions involved or when the Alphabetic Index so directs. Multiple codes should not be used when the classification provides a combination code that clearly identifies all of the elements documented in the diagnosis. When the combination code lacks the necessary specificity to fully describe all elements of a diagnosis, an additional code(s) may be used.

For example, a physician diagnosed a patient who has rheumatoid polyneuropathy as having rheumatoid arthritis of the right ankle and foot. The condition is coded in ICD-10-CM using the combination code. Currently in ICD-9-CM, there is no combination code to fully describe the condition, and two codes must be used for reporting this diagnosis. In ICD-9-CM, this diagnosis would be reported with codes 714.0 (Rheumatoid arthritis) and 351.7 (Polyneuropathy in collagen vascular disease). With ICD-10-CM, a combination code is available, so only one code is reported, M05.571 (Rheumatoid polyneuropathy with rheumatoid arthritis of right ankle and foot). Figure 6.3 illustrates this concept.

FIGURE 6.3 Excerpt From ICD-10-CM

M05.57 Rheumatoid polyneuropathy with rheumatoid arthritis of ankle and foot
Rheumatoid polyneuropathy with rheumatoid arthritis, tarsus, metatarsus and phalanges

    M05.571 **Rheumatoid polyneuropathy with rheumatoid arthritis of right ankle and foot**

    M05.572 Rheumatoid polyneuropathy with rheumatoid arthritis of left ankle and foot

    M05.579 Rheumatoid polyneuropathy with rheumatoid arthritis of unspecified ankle and foot

---

Laterality

For bilateral sites, the final character of the codes in ICD-10-CM indicates laterality. The right side is always character 1, the left side is character 2. In those cases where a bilateral code is appropriate, the bilateral character is always 3. An unspecified side code is also provided for when the side is not identified in the medical record. The unspecified side is either a character 0 or 9, depending on whether it is a fifth or sixth character.

For example, a patient saw her physician for follow-up for an abscess of a bursa in the left shoulder. The first step in coding this patient encounter using ICD-10-CM is to identify the main term. The main term is *abscess*. Notice in this example that the code selection for an abscess of the bursa is based on laterality and affected area. Also note that there are dashes (-) beside the codes, which indicates that additional characters are required. In the example, the abscess of the bursa is in the left shoulder.

Figure 6.4 is an example of the Alphabetic Index in ICD-10-CM.

FIGURE 6.4 **Excerpt From the Alphabetic Index of ICD-10-CM Tabular List**

Abscess (connective tissue) (embolic) (fistulous) (infective) (metastatic) (multiple) (pernicious) (pyogenic) (septic) L02.91

> **bursa M71.00**
> ankle M71.07-
> elbow M71.02-
> foot M71.07-
> hand M71.04-
> hip M71.05-
> knee M71.06-
> multiple sites M71.09
> pharyngeal J39.1
> **shoulder M71.01-**
> specified site NEC M71.08
> wrist M71.03-
> buttock L02.31

Now review Figure 6.5, an example from the Tabular List.

FIGURE 6.5 **Excerpt From ICD-10-CM Tabular List**

M71 Other bursopathies
Excludes1: bunion (M20.1)
bursitis related to use, overuse or pressure (M70.-)
enthesopathies (M76-M77)
M71.0 Abscess of bursa
Use additional code (B95.-, B96.-) to identify causative organism
M71.00 Abscess of bursa, unspecified site
M71.01 Abscess of bursa, shoulder
M71.011 Abscess of bursa, right shoulder
M71.012 Abscess of bursa, left shoulder
M71.019 Abscess of bursa, unspecified shoulder
M71.02 Abscess of bursa, elbow
M71.021 Abscess of bursa, right elbow
M71.022 Abscess of bursa, left elbow
M71.029 Abscess of bursa, unspecified elbow
M71.03 Abscess of bursa, wrist
M71.031 Abscess of bursa, right wrist
M71.032 Abscess of bursa, left wrist
M71.039 Abscess of bursa, unspecified wrist

FIGURE 6.5 **Excerpt From ICD-10-CM Tabular List** *(continued)*

M71.04	Abscess of bursa, hand	
	M71.041	Abscess of bursa, right hand
	M71.042	Abscess of bursa, left hand
	M71.049	Abscess of bursa, unspecified hand
M71.05	Abscess of bursa, hip	
	M71.051	Abscess of bursa, right hip
	M71.052	Abscess of bursa, left hip
	M71.059	Abscess of bursa, unspecified hip
M71.06	Abscess of bursa, knee	
	M71.061	Abscess of bursa, right knee
	M71.062	Abscess of bursa, left knee
	M71.069	Abscess of bursa, unspecified knee
M71.07	Abscess of bursa, ankle and foot	
	M71.071	Abscess of bursa, right ankle and foot
	M71.072	Abscess of bursa, left ankle and foot
	M71.079	Abscess of bursa, unspecified ankle and foot
M71.08	Abscess of bursa, other site	
M71.09	Abscess of bursa, multiple sites	

The correct code selection is M71.012 for this patient encounter. Code M71.01 requires the sixth character, which identifies the laterality of the bursa.

GUIDELINE TIP

When laterality is coded, the right side is always character 1, the left side is character 2, and bilateral is always character 3. The unspecified side is either 0 or 9.

Selection of Principal or First Listed Diagnosis

The code sequenced first on a medical record at the end of an encounter is most important because it defines the main reason for the encounter, as determined at the end of the encounter. In the inpatient setting, the first code listed on a medical record is referred to as the principal diagnosis. In all other health care settings, it is referred to as the first listed code.

The Uniform Hospital Discharge Data Set (UHDDS) definition is, "that condition established after study to be chiefly responsible for occasioning the admission of the patient to the hospital for care." This information can be found in the *Federal Register* (Volume 50, No. 147, pp. 31038-40) published July 31, 1985.

Selection of principal diagnosis/first listed code is based first on the conventions in the classification that provides sequencing instructions. If no sequencing instructions apply, then sequencing is based on the condition(s) that brought the patient into the hospital or physician office and the condition that was the primary focus of treatment.

Conditions present on admission for which the patient is treated but that do not meet the definition of principal diagnosis should be coded as additional codes.

Acute Manifestation Versus Underlying Condition

With the UHDDS definition of principal diagnosis, it is generally an underlying condition that precipitates the need for an admission, because treatment of the underlying condition generally resolves any associated acute manifestations and is the primary focus of treatment. If the acute manifestation is immediately life threatening, and primary treatment is directed at the acute manifestation, the acute manifestation should be sequenced before the underlying condition. If the acute manifestation is not the primary focus of treatment, the underlying condition should be sequenced first.

For example, a patient was treated by his primary care physician for impetigo resulting in otitis externa. The underlying condition is the impetigo, and the manifestation in this example is the otitis externa. This guideline is also based on the fact that the classification has the etiology/manifestation convention that requires the underlying etiology take sequencing precedence over the acute manifestation. Figure 6.6 is an excerpt from the Tabular List.

> **GUIDELINE TIP**
>
> If the acute manifestation is not the primary focus of treatment, the underlying condition should be sequenced first.

FIGURE 6.6 **Excerpt From ICD-10-CM Tabular List**

L01 Impetigo
    Excludes1: impetigo herpetiformis (L40.1)
    L01.0   Impetigo
          Impetigo contagiosa
          Impetigo vulgaris
        L01.00   **Impetigo, unspecified**
               Impetigo NOS
        L01.01   Non-bullous impetigo
        L01.02   Bockhart's impetigo
               Impetigo follicularis
               Perifolliculitis NOS
               Superficial pustular perifolliculitis
        L01.03   Bullous impetigo
               Impetigo neonatorum
               Pemphigus neonatorum
        L01.09   Other impetigo
               Ulcerative impetigo

Code L01.00 (Impetigo, unspecified) is selected as the first listed diagnosis, because in the documentation the type of impetigo is not specified. The secondary diagnosis that should be reported is the otitis externa, code H62.41 (Otitis externa in other diseases classified elsewhere, right ear). Review Figure 6.7.

FIGURE 6.7 **Excerpt From ICD-10-CM Tabular List**

H62 Disorders of external ear in diseases classified elsewhere

    H62.4   Otitis externa in other diseases classified

            H62.40   Otitis externa in other diseases classified elsewhere, unspecified ear

            H62.41   **Otitis externa in other diseases classified elsewhere, right ear**

            H62.42   Otitis externa in other diseases classified elsewhere, left ear

            H62.43   Otitis externa in other diseases classified elsewhere, bilateral

---

Two or More Diagnoses That Equally Meet the Definition of Principal Diagnosis/First Listed Diagnosis

There may be instances when two or more confirmed diagnoses equally meet the criteria for principal/first listed diagnosis as determined by the circumstances of admission, diagnostic workup and/or therapy provided, and sequencing directions are not provided in the Alphabetic Index, Tabular List, or coding guidelines. In this situation, any one of the diagnoses may be sequenced first. This rule applies to the inpatient and outpatient setting.

Original Treatment Plan Not Carried Out

If anticipated treatment is not carried out as a result of unforeseen circumstances, the principal diagnosis/first listed code remains the condition or diagnosis that was planned to be treated.

Complications of Surgery and Other Medical Care

When the patient admission is for treatment of a complication resulting from surgery or other medical care, the complication code is sequenced as the first listed code. If the complication is classified in the category T80-T88 series of codes (Complication of surgical and medical care, not elsewhere classified), an additional code for the specific complication should be assigned if the complication code lacks the necessary specificity in describing the complication.

For example, Dr. Smith performed a spinal puncture on Mr. Cartwright. The patient was doing well following surgery, but later in the evening, the patient was experiencing weakness and a loss of consciousness. The patient was rushed to the emergency department, and Dr. Smith met him there. The physician examined the patient and determined that cerebrospinal fluid was leaking from the puncture site. The physician took the patient into a surgery suite and stopped the leak. The correct code to report would be G97.0 (Cerebrospinal fluid leak from spinal puncture).

FIGURE 6.8 **Excerpt From ICD-10-CM Tabular List**

G97 Intraoperative and postprocedural complications and disorders of nervous system, not elsewhere classified

Excludes2: intraoperative and postprocedural cerebrovascular infarction (I97.81–I97.82-)

G97.0   Cerebrospinal fluid leak from spinal puncture

G97.1   Other reaction to spinal and lumbar puncture

Selection of Secondary Diagnoses

In most cases, more than one code is necessary to fully explain a health care encounter. Though a patient has an encounter for a primary reason (the principal/first listed diagnosis), the additional conditions or reasons for the encounter also need to be coded. These codes are referred to as secondary, additional, or *other* diagnoses. The definition of *other diagnoses* is interpreted as conditions affecting patient care requiring:

- clinical evaluation;
- therapeutic treatment;
- diagnostic procedures;
- extended length of hospital stay; or
- increased nursing care and/or monitoring.

> **GUIDELINE TIP**
>
> When the attending physician includes a diagnosis in the discharge summary or face sheet, it is ordinarily coded unless the condition does not meet the *other diagnosis* definition.

The UHDDS defines *other diagnoses* as "all conditions that coexist at the time of admission, that develop subsequently, or that affect the treatment received and/or the length of stay. Diagnoses that relate to an earlier episode that have no bearing on the current hospital stay are to be excluded" (*ICD-10-CM Official Guidelines for Coding and Reporting*, 2009; page 83). UHDDS definitions apply to inpatients in an acute care, short-term care, and hospital setting. This definition also applies to outpatient encounters.

Previous Conditions

Some physicians include in the diagnostic statement resolved conditions or diagnoses and previous procedures that have no bearing on the current treatment. Such conditions are not to be reported and are coded only if required by practice policy.

For example, a patient was being treated during an encounter for hypertension and diabetes. The patient had pneumonia, which was resolved three months earlier and had no bearing on the services rendered at the visit, so the pneumonia would not be reported with the current encounter.

Abnormal Test Findings

Abnormal test findings (laboratory, radiographic, pathologic, and other diagnostic results) are not coded and reported unless the physician indicates their clinical significance. If the findings are outside the normal range, and the physician has ordered other tests to evaluate the condition or prescribed treatment, it is appropriate to ask the physician whether the abnormal finding should be added.

If the abnormal test finding corresponds to a confirmed diagnosis, it should not be coded in addition to the confirmed diagnosis. A sign or symptom code is to be used as principal/first listed if no definitive diagnosis is established at the time of coding. If the diagnosis is confirmed (eg, a radiograph confirms a fracture, a pathology or laboratory report confirms a diagnosis) prior to coding of the encounter, the confirmed diagnosis code should be used.

Chapter-Specific Guidelines

ICD-10-CM is similar to ICD-9-CM in that it has guidelines for specific diagnoses and/or conditions based on the classification. These guidelines apply to both inpatient and outpatient settings unless indicated. ICD-9-CM has chapter-specific guidelines, and draft guidelines have been created for ICD-10-CM.

Chapter 1 – Certain Infectious and Parasitic Diseases

Chapter 1 (Certain infectious and parasitic diseases) includes guidelines for human immunodeficiency virus, sepsis, infectious agent as the cause of the diseases classified to other chapters, and nosocomial infections.

HIV Guideline 1.1—Human immunodeficiency virus (HIV) diseases

In ICD-10-CM, there is a subcategory with four codes to classify HIV diseases:
- B20   HIV disease
- Z21   Asymptomatic HIV infection status
- R75   Inconclusive laboratory evidence of HIV
- Z20.6 Exposure to HIV.

One complication subcategory exists for HIV complicating pregnancy, childbirth, and the puerperium—subcategory O98.7-.

Category B20 is for use for symptomatic HIV patients when the patient has had any of the infections that are associated with HIV. The code for HIV is synonymous with the term *acquired immune deficiency syndrome* (AIDS) and the AIDS-related complex.

Review the following code example:

B20   HIV disease
      Includes: AIDS, AIDS-related complex, HIV infection, symptomatic
      Use additional code(s) to identify all manifestations of HIV
         infection.
      Excludes1: asymptomatic HIV infection status (Z21), exposure to
         HIV (Z20.6), inconclusive serologic evidence of HIV (R75)

Currently in ICD-9-CM, the appropriate code for a symptomatic HIV patient is 042 (HIV), adding an additional diagnosis code to identify the manifestations of the disease.

People with HIV can get many infections (called *opportunistic infections*). Code Z21 is used for reporting a patient who is diagnosed with HIV-positive status but has never had any related HIV infections. Once a patient has had an HIV-related infection, that patient is assigned code B20 thereafter. The ICD-10-CM official guidelines indicate that a patient should never be assigned R75 or Z21 code, even if at a particular encounter no infection or HIV-related condition is present. Codes B20 and Z21 should never appear on the same record.

Confirmation of HIV status does not require documentation of positive serology or culture for HIV. Reporting is based on the physician's documentation that the patient has an HIV-related illness or is HIV positive.

Review the following ICD-10-CM example:

> **Z21**   Asymptomatic HIV infection status
>   Includes: HIV positive NOS
>   Excludes1: AIDS (B20), contact with or exposure to HIV, (Z20.6),
>   HIV disease (B20), inconclusive laboratory evidence of
>   HIV (R75)

Code Z20.6 is reported only when a patient believes he/she has been exposed to or has come into contact with HIV. The map from ICD-9-CM code V08 (Asymptomatic HIV infection to status) to ICD-10-CM is Z21.

Review the following coding example:

> **Z20.6**   Contact with and exposure to HIV
>   Excludes1: asymptomatic HIV infection status (Z21)

The map from the ICD-9-CM code for HIV exposure, V01.79, to ICD-10-CM is Z20.6.

Code R75 is used when a patient has an inconclusive laboratory test finding for HIV. This code is reported for newborns of HIV-positive mothers whose HIV status has not been confirmed.

Review the following coding example:

> **R75**   Inconclusive laboratory evidence of HIV
>   Includes: nonconclusive HIV-test finding in infants
>   Excludes1: asymptomatic HIV infection status (Z21),
>   HIV disease (B20)

The map from the ICD-9-CM code for inconclusive laboratory evidence of HIV, 797.71, to ICD-10-CM is R75.

The last code related to HIV is 098.7 HIV disease complicating pregnancy, childbirth, and the puerperium. Notice in the example, the specificity of the subcategory is six digits, beginning with the letter O. Diagnosis code O98.71x is reported based on the trimester of pregnancy, whereas O98.72 is reported for

HIV disease complicating childbirth, and O98.72 is reported for complications of the puerperium.

Please note that when a patient has HIV and is pregnant, codes from Chapter 15 of ICD-10-CM, Pregnancy, childbirth, and the puerperium are always sequenced first. Code O98.7- should be sequenced second, followed by the appropriate HIV code.

Review the following example of code 098.7-:

O98.7   HIV disease complicating pregnancy, childbirth, and the puerperium
Use additional code to identify the type of HIV disease:
AIDS (B20)
Asymptomatic HIV status (Z21)
HIV positive NOS (Z21)
Symptomatic HIV disease (B20)

O98.71   HIV disease complicating pregnancy
O98.711   HIV disease complicating pregnancy, first trimester
O98.712   HIV disease complicating pregnancy, second trimester
O98.713   HIV disease complicating pregnancy, third trimester
O98.719   HIV disease complicating pregnancy, unspecified trimester

O98.72   HIV disease complicating childbirth

O98.73   HIV disease complicating the puerperium

Sequencing HIV codes in ICD-10-CM is similar to that in ICD-9-CM. Code B20 should be sequenced as the first listed diagnosis when the patient is treated for an HIV-related condition. Any nonrelated conditions may also be sequenced following the related conditions. When an HIV patient is treated for an unrelated condition, the diagnosis code for the unrelated condition is listed first followed by the HIV-related diagnosis code, which is either B20 for a symptomatic patient or Z21 for an asymptomatic patient.

> **GUIDELINE TIP**
>
> Code B20 should be sequenced as the first listed diagnosis when the patient is treated for an HIV-related condition.

Sepsis and Systemic Inflammatory Response Syndrome

Sepsis refers to an infection due to any organism that triggers a systemic inflammatory response (SIRS). All codes with sepsis in the title include the concept of SIRS. For cases of sepsis that do not result in any associated organ dysfunction, a single code for the type of sepsis should be used.

For other infections in which SIRS is present but sepsis is not in the code title, code R65.1; SIRS may also be assigned. For any infection, if associated organ dysfunction is present, a code from subcategory R65.2, Severe sepsis, should be used, and the guidelines for coding of severe sepsis should be followed. Codes for sepsis and septic shock associated with abortion, ectopic pregnancy, and molar pregnancy are in Chapter 15. Code R65.1 and a code from R65.2 should not be used together on the same record. If a causal organism is not documented, report A41.9, sepsis unspecified for reporting the infection.

Review the following ICD-10-CM example of SIRS and sepsis:

R65.1   Systemic Inflammatory Response Syndrome (SIRS) of non-infectious origin

Excludes1: Sepsis–code to infection

Severe sepsis (R65.2)

R65.2   Severe sepsis infection with organ dysfunction.

Code first underlying condition. Use additional code to identify specific organ dysfunction, such as:

N 17.-	Acute renal failure
N96.0.-	Acute respiratory failure
JG72.81	Critical illness myopathy
G62.81	Critical illness polyneuropathy
D65	Disseminated intravascular coagulopathy [DIC]
G93.41	Encephalopathy (metabolic) (septic)
K72.0-	Hepatic failure

R65.20   Severe sepsis without septic shock

Severe sepsis NOS

R65.21   Severe sepsis with septic shock

The terms *bacteremia* and *septicemia* NOS are coded to R78.81. If a patient with a serious infection is documented to have septicemia, the physician should be asked if the patient has sepsis. If any organ dysfunction is documented, the physician should be asked if the patient has severe sepsis. Negative or inconclusive blood cultures do not preclude a diagnosis of sepsis in patients with clinical evidence of the condition.

R78.8   Finding of other specified substances, not normally found in blood

R78.81   Bacteremia

Septicemia NOS

Excludes1: Sepsis–code to specified infection (A00-B99)

GUIDELINE TIP

The term *urosepsis* is a non-specific term. If the term is used in a medical record, the physician should be asked for which specific condition the term is being used.

Infectious Agents as the Cause of Diseases Classified to Other Chapters

Certain infections are classified in chapters other than Chapter 1, and no organism is identified as part of the infection code. In these instances, it is necessary to use an additional code from Chapter 1 to identify the organism. A code from category B95 (Streptococcus, staphylococcus, and enterococcus as the cause of diseases classified to other chapters), B96 (Other bacterial agents as the cause of diseases classified to other chapters), or B97 (Viral agents as the cause of diseases classified to other chapters) is to be used as an additional code to identify the organism. An instructional note will be found at the infection code advising that an additional organism code is required.

Nosocomial Infections

Nosocomial infections are those that originate or occur in a hospital or hospital-like setting. Nosocomial infections are responsible for about 20,000 deaths in the United States per year. Approximately 10% of American hospital patients (about 2 million every year) acquire a clinically significant nosocomial infection.

If a patient contracts an infection while in the hospital, assign code Y95 (Nosocomial condition) in addition to the diagnosis code for the infection code to identify the infection as nosocomially acquired. ICD-10-CM code Y95 is a three-digit classification.

Chapter 2 – Neoplasms

Neoplasm Table

ICD-10-CM Chapter 2 contains codes for most benign and malignant neoplasms. For proper coding of neoplasms, the documentation in the medical record must indicate that the neoplasm is benign, in situ, malignant, or of uncertain histologic behavior. If there is a malignancy, the secondary (metastatic) site should also be reported, as it is currently with ICD-9-CM.

As in ICD-9-CM, there is a separate Table of Neoplasms. The codes should be selected from the table. The guidelines in ICD-10-CM state, "If the histology (cell type) of the neoplasm is documented, that term should be referenced first, in the main section of the Index, rather than going immediately to the Neoplasm Table, in order to determine which column in the Neoplasm Table is appropriate" (*ICD-10-CM Official Guidelines for Coding and Reporting*, 2009; Chapter 2, Neoplasms, page 21).

For example, a physician diagnosed a 54-year-old female patient with adenocarcinoma of the right breast, lower outer quadrant of the left side. The physician's documentation indicated it as the primary site. The Alphabetic Index should be reviewed prior to referencing the Neoplasm Table. The listing in the Alphabetic Index is "Adenocarcinoma (M8140/3)—see also Neoplasm, malignant." The Alphabetic Index identifies adenocarcinoma as a malignancy reported by site. The coder then will reference the Neoplasm Table for selection of the correct code.

Review Figure 6.9, Neoplasm Table excerpt.

FIGURE 6.9 Excerpt From Neoplasm Table ICD-10-CM

	Malignant Primary	Malignant Secondary	Ca in situ	Benign	Uncertain	Unspecified Behavior
breast (connective tissue)(glandular tissue) (soft parts)						
female						
areola	C50.01-	C79.81	D05.9-	D24.0-	D48.6-	D49.3
axillary tail	C50.61-	C79.81	D05.9-	D24.0-	D48.6-	D49.3
central portion	C50.11-	C79.81	D05.9-	D24.0-	D48.6-	D49.3
inner	C50.81-	C79.81	D05.9-	D24.0-	D48.6-	D49.3
lower	C50.81-	C79.81	D05.9-	D24.0-	D48.6-	D49.3
lower-inner quandrant	C50.31-	C79.81	D05.9-	D24.0-	D48.6-	D49.3
lower-outer quandrant	C50.51-	C79.81	D05.9-	D24.0-	D48.6-	D49.3
mastectomy site (skin)	C44.52	C79.2	-	-	-	-
specified as breast tissue	C50.81-	C79.81	-	-	-	-
midline	C50.81-	C79.81	D05.9-	D24.0-	D48.6-	D49.3
nipple	C50.01-	C79.81	D05.9-	D24.0-	D48.6-	D49.3
outer	C50.81-	C79.81	D05.9-	D24.0-	D48.6-	D49.3
overlapping lesion	C50.81-	-	-	-	-	-
skin	C44.52	C79.2	D04.5	D23.5	D48.5	D49.2
tail (axillary)	C50.61-	C79.81	D05.9-	D24.0-	D48.6-	D49.3
unspecified site	C50.91-	C79.81	D05.9-	D24.0-	D48.6-	D49.3
upper	C50.81-	C79.81	D05.9-	D24.0-	D48.6-	D49.3
upper-inner quandrant	C50.21	C79.81	D05.9-	D24.0-	D48.6-	D49.3
upper-outer quandrant	C50.41-	C79.81	D05.9-	D24.0-	D48.6-	D49.3
male						
areola	C50.02-	C79.81	D05.9-	D24.1-	D48.6-	D49.3
axillary tail	C50.62-	C79.81	D05.9-	D24.1-	D48.6-	D49.3
central portion	C50.12-	C79.81	D05.9-	D24.1-	D48.6-	D49.3
inner	C50.82-	C79.81	D05.9-	D24.1-	D48.6-	D49.3
lower	C50.82-	C79.81	D05.9-	D24.1-	D48.6-	D49.3
lower-inner quandrant	C50.32-	C79.81	D05.9-	D24.1-	D48.6-	D49.3
lower-outer quandrant	C50.52-	C79.81	D05.9-	D24.1-	D48.6-	D49.3
mastectomy site (skin)	C44.52	C79.2	-	-	-	-
specified as breast tissue	C50.82-	C79.81	-	-	-	-
midline	C50.82-	C79.81	D05.9-	D24.1-	D48.6-	D49.3

The correct diagnosis code for this example is C50.52 (Adenocarcinoma of the left side, lower outer quadrant, malignant, primary site), which is found in the first column.

The Neoplasm Table provides proper coding based on the histology of the neoplasm by site. The Tabular List should be referenced to verify that the correct code has been selected and a more specific code does not exist.

Review the Tabular List example in Figure 6.10.

FIGURE 6.10 **Example of a Tabular List**	
C50.51	Malignant neoplasm of lower-outer quadrant of female breast, unspecified side
	C50.511 Malignant neoplasm of lower-outer quadrant of right female breast
	C50.512 Malignant neoplasm of lower-outer quadrant of left female breast
	C50.519 Malignant neoplasm of female breast, unspecified

The guidelines for ICD-10-CM indicate that a confirmed malignancy diagnosis is not reported without a pathology report on the record to confirm the histologic type of neoplasm. If the pathology report is not in the medical record, the attending physician must confirm the diagnosis in the medical record documentation. The pathology report is not required for encounters such as chemotherapy or radiation therapy.

Morphology Codes

The type of histologic tumor is identified with a morphology code. The Neoplasm Table distinguishes only between malignant, benign, in situ, and uncertain behavior. The morphology code should be included in the medical record, when possible. The morphology code can be referenced in the Alphabetic Index under the term for the histology of the neoplasm. This is especially important in coding for the cancer registry.

Neoplasms of Uncertain Behavior Versus Unspecified Behavior

A neoplasm of unspecified behavior is coded in category D49 and is used only when documentation does not exist in the medical record to indicate the nature of the neoplasm. If a histologic examination of the specimen was performed, the unspecified behavior code should not be used.

Code categories D37 to D48 include neoplasms of uncertain behavior, for cases in which, after histologic examination, the pathologist is unable to classify the specimen as benign or malignant, or the cell type cannot be determined.

Sequencing of Neoplasm Codes

If the reason for the encounter is diagnosis of a suspicious lump, skin lesion, or other indication that a malignancy might be present, assign the code for the sign or symptom until confirmation of the diagnosis is made. At the time of coding, if confirmation of a malignancy has been made for an outpatient visit, the neoplasm code should be assigned.

For example, during a routine examination, a physician found a suspicious breast mass in left breast of a female patient who had a history of breast cancer of the right breast. The physician scheduled a biopsy in the outpatient ambulatory surgery center at the hospital. Because the diagnosis of a malignancy could not be confirmed at that visit, the breast mass was reported. In ICD-9-CM, code 611.72 (Lump or mass in breast) would be reported. In ICD-10-CM, code N63 (Unspecified lump in breast, Includes: nodule(s) NOS in breast) would be reported.

If the reason for the encounter is treatment of the primary neoplasm, assign the neoplasm as the principal/first listed diagnosis. The primary site is to be sequenced first, followed by any metastatic sites.

For example, a patient underwent removal of the upper lobe of the lung because of lung cancer after a mass was discovered during a computed tomography scan. The codes are as follows:

ICD-9-CM:　　**162**　　Malignant neoplasm of bronchus or lung
　　　　　　　162.3　Malignant neoplasm of upper lobe, bronchus, or lung

ICD-10-CM:　**C34.1**　Malignant neoplasm of upper lobe, bronchus, or lung
　　　　　　　C34.10　Malignant neoplasm of upper lobe, bronchus, or lung, unspecified side
　　　　　　　C34.11　Malignant neoplasm of upper lobe, right bronchus, or lung
　　　　　　　C34.12　Malignant neoplasm of upper lobe, left bronchus, or lung

The correct ICD-10-CM diagnosis code selection would be C34.10, because the side is not specified. Documentation in this example is extremely important as one can see, because the specificity in the documentation would indicate either the left or right lobe. It is important to begin encouraging physicians to document details more specifically so that the most appropriate diagnosis code can be selected. ICD-10-CM specifies the side of the bronchus or lung; ICD-9-CM does not have this level of specificity.

When an encounter is for a primary malignancy with metastasis, and treatment is directed toward the metastatic (secondary) site(s) only, the metastatic site(s) is/are designated as the principal/first listed diagnosis. The primary malignancy is coded as an additional code.

For example, a patient was diagnosed with a malignant cancer of the pancreatic duct with metastasis to the liver. The patient was being treated for the liver malignancy. The codes are as follows:

ICD-9-CM: First listed diagnosis–197.7　　　Secondary malignant neoplasm of liver

Primary Malignancy–157.3　　　　　　　　Malignant neoplasm of pancreatic duct

ICD-10-CM: First listed diagnosis–C78.7　　Secondary malignant neoplasm of liver

Primary Malignancy–C25.3　　　　　　　　Malignant neoplasm of pancreatic duct

When an encounter is for management of a complication associated with the malignancy, such as dehydration, and the treatment is for the complication only, the complication is coded first, followed by the appropriate code(s) for the malignancy.

For example, a patient was admitted to the hospital after chemotherapy for a malignancy to the ethmoidal sinus. The codes are as follows:

ICD-10-CM: First listed diagnosis–E86.0   Dehydration
Secondary diagnosis–C31.1   Malignant neoplasm of
                                         ethmoidal sinus

An exception to this is anemia due to a neoplasm. Code D63.0 (Anemia in neoplastic disease) is a manifestation (secondary) code. Coding conventions require that it be sequenced after the underlying neoplasm code.

For example, a patient was diagnosed with a malignant neoplasm of the frontal lobe of the brain. The patient was also anemic because of the tumor. See Figure 6.11.

FIGURE 6.11 Excerpt From ICD-10-CM Tabular List, D63

D63 Anemia in chronic diseases classified elsewhere
     D63.0   Anemia in neoplastic disease
              Code first neoplasm (C00-D49)

Two codes are required in this example—the code for the neoplasm and the code for the anemia. Instructional notes identify that the neoplasm is coded first:

First listed diagnosis–C71.1   Malignant neoplasm of frontal lobe
Secondary diagnosis–D63.0   Anemia in neoplastic disease

When an encounter is for a pathological fracture due to a malignancy, if the focus of treatment is the fracture, a code from subcategory M84.5 (Pathological fracture of bone in neoplastic disease) should be sequenced first, followed by the code for the malignancy.

If the focus of treatment is the neoplasm with an associated pathological fracture, the neoplasm code should be sequenced first, followed by a code from M84.5 for the pathological fracture. The *code also* note at M84.5 provides this sequencing instruction.

For example, a patient is treated for a pathologic fracture of the right tibia, resulting from a neoplasm of the right tibia. The first listed diagnosis would be M84.561 followed by the code for the neoplasm.

Review Figure 6.12 from the ICD-10-CM Tabular List.

FIGURE 6.12 Excerpt From ICD-10-CM Tabular List, M84.5

M84.5 Pathologic fracture of bone in neoplastic disease
    Code also underlying neoplasm
    The following seventh character extensions are to be added to each code for subcategory M84.5:
    A initial encounter for fracture
    D subsequent encounter for fracture with routine healing
    G subsequent encounter for fracture with delayed healing
    K subsequent encounter for fracture with nonunion
    P subsequent encounter for fracture with malunion
    S sequela

    M84.561a   Pathologic fracture of bone in neoplastic disease, right tibia

---

The codes would be reported in the following sequence:

First listed diagnosis–M84.561A   Pathologic fracture of bone in neoplastic disease, right tibia
Secondary diagnosis–C76.51   Malignant neoplasm of right lower limb

The seventh character, *a*, identifies the initial patient encounter for the condition.

When an encounter is for pain management due to a malignancy, the pain code G89.3 should be sequenced first, followed by the appropriate neoplasm code(s).

For example, a patient with a malignancy of the frontal lobe of the brain was in acute pain during his follow-up visit. The physician prescribed a drug to relieve the patient's pain. The codes are as follows:

First listed diagnosis–G89.3   Neoplasm related pain (acute) (chronic)
    Code also neoplasm
Secondary diagnosis–C71.1   Malignant neoplasm of frontal lobe

When the reason for the patient encounter is management of the neoplasm and the pain is associated with the neoplasm, code G89.3 may be assigned as an additional diagnosis. It is not necessary to code the site of the pain in this instance.

When the encounter is for treatment of a complication resulting from a surgical procedure performed for the treatment of a malignancy, designate the complication as the principal/first listed diagnosis if treatment is directed at resolving the complication.

For example, a patient was treated for sepsis following surgery for the removal of a malignant tumor of the lateral wall of the bladder. The codes are as follows:

First listed diagnosis–T81.4xxA   Infection following a procedure, not
                                   elsewhere classified; Sepsis following a
                                   procedure, not elsewhere classified
Secondary diagnosis–C67.2   Malignant neoplasm of lateral wall of
                                   bladder

Tabular List note:
The following seventh character extensions are to be added to
each code for category T81:
                                   A initial encounter
                                   D subsequent encounter
                                   S sequela

The seventh character extension is A for the initial patient encounter for the
sepsis. Two dummy "x" placeholders must be added to the code since the code
T81.4 has only four characters, and the code requires the seventh character
extension.

When a primary malignancy has been previously excised or eradicated from
its site, and there is no further treatment directed to that site, and there is no evidence of any existing primary malignancy, a code from category Z85.- (Personal
history of primary and secondary malignant neoplasm) should be used to indicate the former site of the malignancy if no related pathology is discovered.

Any mention of extension, invasion, or metastasis to another site(s) is coded
as a secondary malignant neoplasm to the metastatic site(s). The secondary site
may be the principal/first listed, with the Z85 code used as a secondary code.

For example, a 56-year-old male was seen in follow-up following removal of the
prostate gland three years earlier for a malignancy. The diagnosis code reported
is Z85.46 (Personal history of primary malignant neoplasm of prostate).

When a primary malignancy has been excised, but further treatment, such
as additional surgery, radiation therapy, or chemotherapy, is directed to that site,
the primary malignancy code, not the Z85 code, should be used until treatment
is completed.

Cancer in a Pregnant Patient

When a patient is treated for a malignant neoplasm that complicates pregnancy,
childbirth, or the puerperium, a code from subcategory O94.1- (Malignant neoplasm complicating pregnancy, childbirth, and the puerperium) should be used
first, followed by the appropriate code to indicate the type of neoplasm.

For example, a 32-year-old patient in the second trimester of pregnancy was
treated by her oncologist for a primary malignancy of the pineal gland.

First listed diagnosis–O9A.112   Malignant neoplasm complicating
                                  pregnancy, second trimester
Secondary diagnosis–C75.3   Malignant neoplasm of the pineal gland

Malignant Neoplasm Without Specification of Site

Code C80.1 (Malignant neoplasm without specification of site) equates to cancer, unspecified. It is also for disseminated cancer for which no primary site is found. This code should be used only when no determination can be made as to the primary site of a malignancy. It should not be used in place of assigning codes for the primary site and for all known secondary sites. The following example is from the Tabular List:

C80 Malignant neoplasm without specification of site
   Excludes1: malignant neoplasm of specified multiple sites–code
    to each site

  C80.0 Disseminated malignant neoplasm, unspecified
    Carcinomatosis NOS
    Generalized cancer, unspecified site (primary) (secondary)
    Generalized malignancy, unspecified site (primary)
     (secondary)

  C80.1 Malignant neoplasm, unspecified
    Cancer unspecified site (primary) (secondary)
    Carcinoma unspecified site (primary) (secondary)
    Malignancy unspecified site (primary) (secondary)

Encounters for Chemotherapy and Radiation Therapy

As with ICD-9-CM, when an encounter involves the surgical removal of a neoplasm, primary or secondary site, followed by chemotherapy or radiation treatment, chemotherapy or radiation therapy diagnosis should be the first listed diagnosis, followed by the malignancy.

If an encounter is solely for the administration of chemotherapy or radiation therapy, code Z51.0 (Encounter for antineoplastic radiation therapy), Z51.11 (Encounter for antineoplastic chemotherapy), or Z51.12 (Encounter for antineoplastic immunotherapy) should be reported as the first listed or principal diagnosis.

When a patient receives both chemotherapy and radiation therapy, both codes should be listed in either order of sequence.

For example, a patient underwent chemotherapy following an oophorectomy for removal of a malignant tumor of the left ovary. The codes are as follows:

First listed diagnosis–Z51.11 Encounter for chemotherapy for the malignant tumor of the left ovary
Secondary diagnosis–C56.1 Malignant neoplasm of left ovary

When an encounter is for the purpose of radiotherapy or chemotherapy, and the patient develops such complications as uncontrolled nausea and vomiting or dehydration, the principal/first listed code remains the radiation therapy or chemotherapy code. The complications of the treatment should be added as additional codes following the code(s) for the malignancy.

For example, a patient was experiencing nausea and vomiting following radiation therapy for treatment of a malignant tumor of the parathyroid gland. The codes are as follows:

First listed diagnosis–Z51.0	Encounter for radiotherapy session
Secondary diagnosis–C75.0	Malignant neoplasm of parathyroid gland
Tertiary diagnosis–R11.0	Nausea with vomiting

When an encounter is to determine the extent of the malignancy or for a procedure to treat the malignancy, the primary malignancy or appropriate metastatic site is designated as the principal/first listed diagnosis even if chemotherapy or radiotherapy is administered.

For example, a physician removed a malignant tumor from the descending colon in the outpatient surgery center. The physician recommended that the patient undergo chemotherapy the same day. The codes are as follows:

First listed diagnosis–C18.6	Malignant neoplasm of descending colon
Secondary diagnosis–Z51.11	Chemotherapy session for neoplasm

When an encounter is for management of a complication of chemotherapy or radiation therapy, and the only treatment is for the complication, the complication is sequenced first, followed by the appropriate code(s) for the malignancy.

For example, a patient was experiencing nausea and vomiting one day after chemotherapy to treat the left breast. The codes are as follows:

First listed diagnosis–R11.0	Nausea with vomiting
Secondary diagnosis–C50.312	Malignant neoplasm of lower-inner quadrant of left female breast

Because of the potentially toxic nature of many chemotherapy agents, certain tests may be performed prior to the administration of chemotherapy as well as during the course of the chemotherapy treatment. The malignancy should be coded as the principal diagnosis for encounters for these tests.

GUIDELINE TIP

Code neoplasms using the Neoplasm Table, and verify the code with the Tabular List in ICD-10-CM.

Endocrine Therapy

Endocrine therapy such as tamoxifen may be given prophylactically for women at high risk of developing breast cancer. It may also be given during cancer treatment as well as following treatment to help prevent recurrence. The use of endocrine therapy does not affect the guidelines for coding of neoplasms.

Chapter 3 – Diseases of the Blood and Blood-Forming Organs and Certain Disorders Involving the Immune Mechanism

There are no specific chapter guidelines in this chapter, and it is reserved for future guideline expansion. Chapter guidelines for this chapter may be added prior to final implementation.

Chapter 4 – Endocrine, Nutritional, and Metabolic Diseases

Within this category are the following blocks:
- E00–E07   Disorders of thyroid gland
- E08–E13   Diabetes mellitus
- E15–E16   Other disorders of glucose regulation and pancreatic internal secretion
- E20–E35   Disorders of other endocrine glands
- E36   Intraoperative complications of endocrine system
- E40–E46   Malnutrition
- E50–E64   Other nutritional deficiencies
- E65–E68   Overweight, obesity, and other hyperalimentation
- E70–E88   Metabolic disorders
- E89   Postprocedural endocrine and metabolic complications and disorders, not elsewhere classified.

The largest change in the guidelines from ICD-9-CM to ICD-10-CM is coding for diabetes mellitus. The diabetes mellitus codes have been expanded in ICD-10-CM to report a higher level of specificity and include the following combination codes:
- Type of diabetes mellitus
- Body system affected
- Complications affecting that body system.

There are five diabetes mellitus categories in the ICD-10-CM. They are:
- E08   Diabetes mellitus due to an underlying condition
- E09   Drug or chemical induced diabetes mellitus
- E10   Type I diabetes mellitus
- E11   Type 2 diabetes mellitus
- E13   Other specified diabetes mellitus.

All these categories, with the exception of E10, include a note directing users to use an additional code to identify any insulin use, which is Z79.4. The concept of *insulin-requiring* and *non-insulin-requiring* is not a component of the diabetes mellitus categories in ICD-10-CM. Code Z79 (long-term current use of insulin) is added to identify the use of insulin for diabetic management even if the patient is not insulin dependent in code categories E08 to E09 and E11 to E13.

The fourth character under these categories refers to underlying conditions with specified complications, whereas the fifth character defines the specific manifestation such as neuropathy or angiopathy.

Definitions for the types of diabetes mellitus are included in the *Includes* notes under each diabetes mellitus category. Diabetes codes from categories E08 to E09 have a *code first* note, indicating that diabetes is to be sequenced after the underlying condition, drug, or chemical that is responsible for the diabetes. Codes from categories E10 to E13 (Diabetes mellitus) are sequenced first, followed by codes for any additional complications outside of these categories, if applicable.

With the exception of category E10, all of the ICD-10-CM categories for diabetes include a note that directs the coder to use an additional code to identify insulin usage (Z79.4). Fourth characters under these categories refer to underlying conditions with specified complications. Fifth characters define the specific manifestation (ie, ketoacidosis, nephropathy, neuropathy, peripheral angiopathy). Sixth characters further define the manifestations.

Consider a type I diabetic patient with Kimmelstiel-Wilson disease who visited his endocrinologist for follow-up. Figure 6.13 compares ICD-9-CM with ICD-10-CM for coding this example.

GUIDELINE TIP

Use an additional code to identify insulin usage (Z79.7), if applicable, when coding diabetes mellitus.

FIGURE 6.13 **Comparison Between ICD-9-CM and ICD-10-CM for Coding of Diabetes**

ICD-9-CM		ICD-10-CM	
250.41	Diabetes with renal manifestations, type I (juvenile type), not stated as uncontrolled	E10.21	Type 1 diabetes mellitus with diabetic nephropathy Type 1 diabetes mellitus with Kimmelstiel-Wilson disease
581.81	Nephropathy, not otherwise specified	E08.21	Diabetes mellitus due to underlying condition with diabetic nephropathy

---

Diabetes Mellitus in Pregnant Patient

Codes for pregnancy, childbirth, and the puerperium, which are located in Chapter 15 of ICD-10-CM, are always sequenced first in the medical record. A patient who has preexisting diabetes mellitus and becomes pregnant should be assigned a code from category O24 (Diabetes mellitus in pregnancy, childbirth, and the puerperium), followed by the diabetes code from Chapter 4 of ICD-10-CM. These codes have been expanded in ICD-10-CM. The fourth character subcategory codes identify the type of diabetes as preexisting type 1 or type 2, unspecified, or gestational.

The fifth character indicates whether the diabetes is treated during pregnancy, childbirth, or the puerperium. The sixth character indicates the trimester during which treatment is sought. With gestational diabetes, the sixth character identifies whether the gestational diabetes is diet controlled, insulin controlled, or whether control is unspecified.

For example, a 25-year-old patient with diabetes mellitus type 1 in the second trimester of pregnancy had a routine visit with her obstetrician. The patient's blood sugar was well controlled, and the patient indicated that she was doing well with her diet and exercise regimen. The physician scheduled the patient for follow-up in one month. Figure 6.14 shows the relevant codes.

FIGURE 6.14 Comparison Between ICD-9-CM and ICD-10-CM for Coding of Diabetes During Pregnancy

ICD-9-CM		ICD-10-CM	
648.03	Maternal diabetes mellitus, antepartum	O24.012	Pre-existing diabetes mellitus, type 1, in pregnancy, second trimester
250.01	Diabetes mellitus without of complication, type I (juvenile type), not stated as uncontrolled	E10.69	Type 1 diabetes mellitus with other specified complication

In another example, a 27-year-old patient developed gestational diabetes in the third trimester of pregnancy. The patient's condition was controlled with diet and exercise. Figure 6.15 shows the relevant codes.

FIGURE 6.15 Comparison Between ICD-9-CM and ICD-10-CM for Coding of Gestational Diabetes

ICD-9-CM		ICD-10-CM	
648.8	Abnormal glucose tolerance Gestational diabetes	O24.41	Gestational diabetes mellitus in pregnancy
	648.83 Abnormal maternal glucose tolerance, antepartum		**O24.410 Gestational diabetes mellitus in pregnancy, diet-controlled**

Diabetic patients who have a pancreatic transplant for treatment of diabetes mellitus may no longer require insulin or other care for their diabetes mellitus, but preexisting complications from the diabetes may still exist after transplant. Codes from the diabetes mellitus categories are still applicable to describe the complication in these cases. A transplant status code should be used with the diabetes code in this circumstance. An example is given in Figure 6.16.

FIGURE 6.16 Comparison Between ICD-9-CM and ICD-10-CM for Coding of Pancreatic Transplant Status

ICD-9-CM		ICD-10-CM	
V42.83	Pancreas replaced by transplant	Z94.83	Pancreas transplant status

Complications due to insulin pump malfunction or failure are assigned a code from subcategory T85.6 (Mechanical complication of other specified internal and external prosthetic devices, implants, and grafts), which identifies the type of pump malfunction. A code from this category is listed as the first listed diagnosis, followed by a code from T38.3x6- to report the underdosing of insulin or oral hypoglycemic agent.

When an insulin pump malfunction results in an overdose of insulin, the first listed diagnosis code is T85.6- (Mechanical complications of other specified internal and external prosthetic devices, implants, or grafts). A secondary code of T38.3x1-[Poisoning by insulin and oral hypoglycemic drugs, accidental (unintentional)] is reported.

Chapter 5 – Mental and Behavioral Disorders

Codes for mental and behavioral disorders in ICD-10-CM range from F01 to F99. These codes are found in Chapter 5 of the ICD-10-CM Tabular List. In most cases, Chapter 5 parallels codes found in the *Diagnostic and Statistical Manual of Mental Disorders* (4th ed), published by the American Psychiatric Association.

This chapter contains the following blocks:
- F01–F09   Mental disorders due to known physiological conditions
- F10–F19   Mental and behavioral disorders due to psychoactive substance use
- F20–F29   Schizophrenia, schizotypal and delusional, and other non-mood psychotic disorders
- F30–F39   Mood (affective) disorders
- F40–F48   Anxiety, dissociative, stress-related, somatoform, and other nonpsychotic mental disorders
- F50–F59   Behavioral syndromes associated with physiological disturbances and physical factors
- F60–F69   Disorders of adult personality and behavior
- F70–F79   Mental retardation
- F80–F89   Pervasive and specific developmental disorders
- F90–F98   Behavioral and emotional disorders with onset usually occurring in childhood and adolescence
- F99   Unspecified mental disorder.

Guidelines for Chapter 5

Assign code F45.41 for pain that is exclusively psychological. There is also, generally, a psychological component of any type of acute or chronic pain.

Code F45.41 (Pain disorder with related psychological factors) should be used following the appropriate code from category G89 (Pain, not elsewhere classified), if there is documentation of a psychological component for a patient with acute or chronic pain.

The drug and alcohol codes are multiaxial, combination codes that identify the substance, the type of use, abuse, or dependence and the complications and manifestations caused by the substance. The category level is the substance, such as alcohol (F10) and other types of drugs (F11-F19), including nicotine (F17).

An instructional note in the Tabular List for F10 is applicable to this category:

Use additional code for blood alcohol level, if applicable (Y90.-)
  F10.1 Alcohol abuse
    Excludes1: alcohol dependence (F10.2-),
      alcohol use, unspecified (F10.9-)

Review the comparison between ICD-9-CM and ICD-10-CM in Figure 6.17.

FIGURE 6.17 Comparison Between ICD-9-CM and ICD-10-CM for Coding of Alcohol Abuse

ICD-9-CM			ICD-10-CM		
305.0		Nondependent alcohol abuse	F10.12		Alcohol abuse with intoxication
	305.00	Nondependent alcohol abuse, unspecified drunkenness		F10.120	Alcohol abuse with intoxication, uncomplicated
	305.01	Nondependent alcohol abuse, continuous drunkenness		F10.121	Alcohol abuse with intoxication delirium
	305.02	Nondependent alcohol abuse, episodic drunkenness		F10.129	Alcohol abuse with intoxication, unspecified
	305.03	Nondependent alcohol abuse, in remission			

The fourth character axis distinguishes abuse or dependence. The fifth and sixth characters indicate the complication, such as withdrawal or delusions. The types of complications and manifestations at the fifth and sixth character level are specific to the type of drug.

Multiple codes from a single category from categories F10 to F19 may be used together if a patient has multiple complications from a single substance. Multiple codes from different categories from F10 to F19 may be used together if a patient has used more than one substance and has multiple complications associated with the use of the substances.

For example, a 26-year-old male was taken to the emergency department by the local sheriff after the patient became disruptive in a local nightclub. The patient tested positive for cocaine, and his blood alcohol level was 0.21. The patient was suffering from alcohol abuse, which was uncomplicated, and cocaine abuse with cocaine-induced mood disorder.

The encounter would be reported with two codes:

F10.120   Alcohol abuse with intoxication, uncomplicated

F14.14   Cocaine abuse with cocaine-induced mood disorder

An additional code from category Y90 (Evidence of alcohol involvement determined by blood alcohol level) should be used with a code from F10 (Alcohol-related disorders) if the patient's blood alcohol level is recorded. A code from Y90 should be recorded only once, at the initial blood alcohol level reading. The codes are as follows:

Y90   Evidence of alcohol involvement determined by blood alcohol level.
　　　Code first any associated alcohol-related disorders (F10)
　　Y90.0   Blood alcohol level of less than 20 mg/100 mL
　　Y90.1   Blood alcohol level of 20-39 mg/100 mL
　　Y90.2   Blood alcohol level of 40-59 mg/100 mL
　　Y90.3   Blood alcohol level of 60-79 mg/100 mL
　　Y90.4   Blood alcohol level of 80-99 mg/100 mL
　　Y90.5   Blood alcohol level of 100-119 mg/100 mL
　　Y90.6   Blood alcohol level of 120-199 mg/100 mL
　　Y90.7   Blood alcohol level of 200-239 mg/100 mL
　　Y90.8   Blood alcohol level of 240 mg/100 mL or more
　　Y90.9   Presence of alcohol in blood, level not specified

In another example, a 22-year-old college student was taken to the emergency department after excessive drinking at a fraternity party. The patient stated that she drank several glasses of wine. The patient complained of headache, excessive vomiting, nausea, fatigue, and loss of memory. A blood test indicated the patient was intoxicated. The physician examined the patient and diagnosed the patient with alcohol abuse, which was uncomplicated, along with dehydration. The patient was given intravenous fluids and released two hours later.

The codes are as follows:

F10.120   Alcohol abuse with intoxication, uncomplicated

Y90.9   Presence of alcohol in blood, level not specified

Codes from the poisoning and toxic effects section of Chapter 19 (T40, T51) should be used in conjunction with the F10 to F19 codes if a patient has acute alcohol or drug poisoning or overdose, even if the patient is dependent on alcohol or drugs.

For example, a patient overdosed on cocaine and was taken by ambulance to the emergency department at a local hospital. The patient was diagnosed with cocaine abuse and cocaine poisoning. The patient indicated this was the first time he had used cocaine. The patient was treated and referred to a drug treatment program.

The patient encounter would be reported as follows:

F14.129   Cocaine abuse with intoxication, unspecified

T40.5x1a   Poisoning by cocaine, accidental (unintentional)
Poisoning by cocaine NOS

Instructional notes for T40 indicate that a seventh character extension is required. The following seventh character extensions are to be added to each code for category T40:

A initial encounter
D subsequent encounter
S sequela.

Notice that the fifth character extension is *x*, which is a dummy placeholder for future expansion.

Dementia with Associated Behavioral Disorders

F02 (Dementia in other diseases classified elsewhere) is a manifestation category that is used with codes for specific types of dementia, such as Alzheimer's disease (G30). The code for the specific type of dementia is sequenced first, followed by the appropriate code from category F02. The code from category F02 indicates whether the dementia has an associated behavioral disturbance.

For example, a patient with Alzheimer's disease living in a nursing home wandered off the premises. The staff notified the police, and the patient was found three hours later unharmed. The patient was taken to the infirmary, where the physician examined the patient before returning her to her room.

The service is reported with two codes. Because the type of dementia is not documented, the diagnosis is reported as Alzheimer's disease, unspecified, with an additional code F02.81 to identify the dementia with the behavioral disturbance. Code F02.81 includes dementia with wandering off.

The patient encounter is reported with the following two diagnoses:

G30.9   Alzheimer's disease, unspecified

F02.81   Dementia in other diseases classified elsewhere, with behavioral disturbance

Dementia in other diseases classified elsewhere with aggressive behavior

Dementia in other diseases classified elsewhere with combative behavior

Dementia in other diseases classified elsewhere with violent behavior

Dementia in other diseases classified elsewhere with wandering off

Chapter 6 – Diseases of the Nervous System

Dominant versus Nondominant Side Guideline

For patients with hemiplegia and other paralytic syndromes, the side involved is important in determining potential for recovery. Patients whose dominant side is affected will have a more difficult time with rehabilitation than patients whose nondominant side is affected. Generally, the patient's side dominance is recorded in the initial history and physical. If there is reference to a patient's being right-handed or left-handed, this indicates dominance. Dominance is present in both the upper and lower limbs.

In ICD-9-CM, hemiplegia is coded as 438.20 or 438.22, using the same criteria for code selection as ICD-10-CM. The exception is the expansion as to the type of hemiplegia, which must be reported.

Codes from category G81 (Hemiplegia and hemiparesis) and subcategories G83.1- (Monoplegia of lower limb), G83.2- (Monoplegia of upper limb), and G83.3- (Monoplegia, unspecified) have a final character for dominant and nondominant side. If the information is not available in the record, the default should be dominant. For ambidextrous patients, the default should also be dominant. Figure 6.18 shows the relevant codes.

FIGURE 6.18 Comparision Between ICD-9-CM and ICD-10-CM for Coding of Hemiplegia

ICD-9-CM			ICD-10-CM	
438.2	Hemiplegia/hemiparesis		G81.00	Flaccid hemiplegia affecting unspecified side
	438.20	Hemiplegia affecting unspecified side	G81.01	Flaccid hemiplegia affecting right dominant side
	438.21	Hemiplegia affecting dominant side due to cerebrovascular disease	G81.02	Flaccid hemiplegia affecting left dominant side
			G81.03	Flaccid hemiplegia affecting right nondominant side
	438.22	Hemiplegia affecting nondominant side due to cerebrovascular disease	G81.04	Flaccid hemiplegia affecting left nondominant side
			G81.1	Spastic hemiplegia
			G81.10	Spastic hemiplegia affecting unspecified side
			G81.11	Spastic hemiplegia affecting right dominant side
			G81.12	Spastic hemiplegia affecting left dominant side
			G81.13	Spastic hemiplegia affecting right nondominant side
			G81.14	Spastic hemiplegia affecting left nondominant side

FIGURE 6.18 **Comparision Between ICD-9-CM and ICD-10-CM for Coding of Hemiplegia** *(continued)*	
ICD-9-CM	**ICD-10-CM**
	G81.9 Hemiplegia, unspecified
	G81.90 Hemiplegia, unspecified affecting unspecified side
	G81.91 Hemiplegia, unspecified affecting right dominant side
	G81.92 Hemiplegia, unspecified affecting left dominant side
	G81.93 Hemiplegia, unspecified affecting right nondominant side
	G81.94 Hemiplegia, unspecified affecting left nondominant side

This category is to be used only when hemiplegia (complete)(incomplete) is reported without further specification or is stated to be old or longstanding but of unspecified cause. The category is also used in multiple coding to identify these types of hemiplegia resulting from any noncongenital, neurologic cause.

Parkinson's Disease

There are two categories in ICD-10-CM for Parkinson's disease—G20 Parkinson's disease and G21 Secondary parkinsonism. Within ICD-10-CM, code G20 is for reporting primary Parkinson's disease. It is the default code for the condition. This category includes the following:

- Hemiparkinsonism
- Idiopathic parkinsonism
- Parkinson's disease paralysis
- Agitans parkinsonism
- Parkinson's disease NOS
- Primary parkinsonism.

Compare ICD-9-CM to ICD-10-CM in Figure 6.19. Notice that the categories are similar.

FIGURE 6.19 **Comparison Between ICD-9-CM and ICD-10-CM for Coding of Parkinson's Disease**

ICD-9-CM		ICD-10-CM	
332	Parkinson's disease	G20	Parkinson's disease
	332.0 Paralysis agitans		Primary
	Primary		Hemiparkinsonism
	Idiopathic		Idiopathic
	NOS		Parkinson's disease paralysis
			Agitans parkinsonism
			Parkinson's disease NOS

Secondary parkinsonism, coded G21., is a result of another condition, such as encephalitis or poisoning. The symptoms of Parkinson's disease develop secondary to the initial condition. The sequencing of a code from G21 is based on the conventions found at the G21 code level.

Category G21 excludes dementia with parkinsonism and is coded G31.83. Instructional notes should be followed for *Excludes1* along with the instruction to code first T36 to T50 to identify drug-induced secondary parkinsonism or external agent(s), using codes T51 to T65.

Compare ICD-9-CM and ICD-10-CM in Figure 6.20 for category G21 in ICD-10-CM and subclassification 332 for Parkinson's disease.

FIGURE 6.20 **Comparison Between ICD-9-CM and ICD-10-CM for Coding of Secondary Parkinson's Disease**

ICD-9-CM		ICD-10-CM		
332	Parkinson's disease	G21	Secondary parkinsonism	
	332.1 Secondary parkinsonism		G21.0 Malignant neuroleptic syndrome	
			G21.1 Other drug-induced secondary parkinsonism	
				G21.11 Neuroleptic induced parkinsonism
			G21.2 Secondary parkinsonism due to other external agents	

The shakes and tremors associated with Parkinson's disease are also symptoms of a form of dementia, dementia with Lewy bodies (G31.83). The term *dementia with Parkinsonism* is included under code G31.83 which is excluded from G21.

Category G31.8 is classified as other specified degenerative diseases of the nervous system. Some codes in this classification are shown in Figure 6.21.

FIGURE 6.21 Excerpt From ICD-10-CM Tabular List, G31.8

G31.8   Other specified degenerative diseases of the nervous system

      G31.81   Alpers' disease

            gray matter degeneration

      G31.82   Leigh's disease

            subacute necrotizing encephalopathy

      G31.83   Dementia with Lewy bodies

            Dementia with parkinsonism

            Lewy body dementia

            Lewy body disease

      G31.84   Mild cognitive impairment, so stated

      G31.89   Other specified degenerative diseases of nervous system

G31.9   Degenerative disease of nervous system, unspecified

For example, a patient diagnosed with dementia with Parkinsonism was transferred from the hospital to the nursing home after discharge. The relevant ICD-9-CM code is 331.82 (Dementia with Lewy bodies), and the relevant ICD-10-CM code is G31.83 (Dementia with Lewy bodies).

Cases of dementia are often diagnosed strictly by the symptoms and behavior of the patient. For certain types of dementia, confirmation of the diagnosis can be made only at autopsy. For this reason, physicians often document probable or suspected dementia. Dementia is one group of conditions in which it is acceptable to code the condition even if it is stated as probable or suspected.

Guidelines for Coding Dementia

In the ICD-10-CM guidelines, two codes are required for dementia. First the dementia is coded, followed by a secondary code from category F02 for the behavioral component of the dementia.

Dementia is classified as other cerebral degenerations in ICD-9-CM. Dementia is a slowly progressing decline in mental ability in which memory, judgment, thinking, the ability to pay attention, and learning are impaired. With some conditions, personality may deteriorate. Dementia usually affects persons over 60 years old, but it can develop suddenly in younger people when brain cells are destroyed by trauma, injury, disease, or toxic substances. Dementia is not a normal process of aging, although as people age they often experience short-term memory loss and a decline in learning ability. Dementia is also possible after brain injury or cardiac arrest when the oxygen supply to the brain has been jeopardized.

For example, a family practitioner examined a 68-year-old female patient. The patient's daughter, who was with her, told the physician that her mother was experiencing episodes of memory loss and loss of orientation to time and place and sometimes does did not know her. The patient had been experiencing these episodes gradually over the previous year, but in the previous two months her condition had worsened. The patient had experienced combative and aggressive behavior for the previous two weeks, which prompted the visit. After examining the patient, the physician explained to the daughter that the patient was experiencing signs of dementia resulting from Alzheimer's disease and would require constant care because her condition was worsening. The diagnosis documented in the medical record was Alzheimer's disease with dementia.

Using ICD-10-CM, two codes are required—one for the Alzheimer's disease with dementia and a secondary code from category F02. Code F02.8 requires a fifth digit extension.

Figures 6.22 and 6.23 illustrate the code choices for category F02.8.

FIGURE 6.22 Excerpt From ICD-10-CM Tabular List, F02.8

F02.8   Dementia in other diseases classified elsewhere

     F02.80   Dementia in other diseases classified elsewhere, without behavioral disturbance

               Dementia in other diseases classified elsewhere NOS

     F02.81   Dementia in other diseases classified elsewhere, with behavioral disturbance

               Dementia in other diseases classified elsewhere with aggressive behavior

               Dementia in other diseases classified elsewhere with combative behavior

               Dementia in other diseases classified elsewhere with violent behavior

               Dementia in other diseases classified elsewhere with wandering off

---

Compare ICD-9-CM with ICD-10-CM coding for Alzheimer's disease.

DOCUMENTATION TIP

Dementia is coded as the principal/first listed diagnosis, followed by a secondary code from category F02 for the behavioral component of the dementia.

FIGURE 6.23 Comparison Between ICD-9-CM and ICD-10-CM for Coding of Alzheimer's Disease

ICD-9-CM		ICD-10-CM	
331.0	Alzheimer's disease (first listed diagnosis)	G30	Alzheimer's disease
294.11	Dementia in conditions classified elsewhere with behavioral disturbance (secondary diagnosis)	G30.9	Alzheimer's disease with behavioral disturbance (first listed diagnosis)
		F02.81	Dementia in other diseases classified elsewhere, with behavioral disturbance (secondary diagnosis)

Pain Management

Category G89 is used for reporting pain management or pain control. The following guidelines in ICD-10-CM are used for this category:

1 When the patient encounter is for pain control, assign G89 followed by the code identifying the site of pain.

2 If the patient encounter is for reasons other than pain control or management and a confirmed diagnosis has not been confirmed by the provider, the code for the specific site of pain is listed first, followed by the appropriate code from category 89.

3 When a neurostimulator is inserted for pain control, assign an appropriate pain code as the first listed diagnosis.

4 When a patient encounter is for treating the underlying condition, and a neurostimulator is inserted for pain control during the same encounter, the code for the underlying condition is assigned as the first listed diagnosis, followed by the diagnosis for the pain.

5 Postoperative pain not associated with a specific complication is assigned the appropriate pain code from category G89.-.

6 When pain is associated with a specific postoperative complication, assign as the first listed diagnosis a code from Chapter 19 (Injury, poisoning, and certain other consequences and external causes), along with an additional code to identify acute or chronic pain, using G89.18 or G89.28.

7 Chronic pain is classified to subcategory G89.2. The provider's documentation should guide the use of these codes, as there is no specific time frame defining when pain becomes chronic.

8 Code G89.3 is reported when pain is associated with a malignancy or tumor, regardless of whether the malignancy is primary or secondary. This code is also assigned whether the pain is acute or chronic.

9   G89.3 is assigned as the first listed diagnosis when the reason for the patient encounter is pain control or management. The neoplasm should be reported as a secondary diagnosis.

10 When the neoplasm is the reason for the patient encounter, and there is documented pain associated with the neoplasm, report G89.3 as an additional diagnosis. The site of the pain is not required for reporting.

11 Central pain syndrome (G89.0) or chronic pain syndrome (G89.4) may be reported when the provider documents this information in the medical record.

For example, a patient suffering from neck pain following a car accident was treated by an orthopedic surgeon for the chronic pain.
Correct diagnosis code reporting is as follows:

First listed diagnosis–G89.11   Acute pain due to trauma
Secondary diagnosis–M54.2   Cervicalgia

In another example, a patient with a malignancy of the frontal lobe of the brain was in acute pain during his follow-up visit. The physician prescribed a drug to relieve the pain. The codes are as follows:

First listed diagnosis–G89.3   Neoplasm-related pain (acute) (chronic)
Secondary diagnosis–C71.1   Malignant neoplasm of frontal lobe

Summary

It is important to understand the ICD-10-CM official guidelines, along with related coding issues, to understand the implementation process. Implementing ICD-10-CM preparation includes an understanding of the ICD-10-CM general guidelines as well as chapter-specific guidelines that the user will be referencing in the migration to ICD-10-CM in every practice, no matter what the specialty.

Resources

ICD-10-CM Official Guidelines for Coding and Reporting, 2009. Available online at ftp://ftp.cdc.gov/pub/Health_Statistics/NCHS/Publications/ICD10CM/2009/.

National Center for Health Statistics. *ICD-10-CM Tabular List.* Available online at ftp://ftp.cdc.gov/pub/Health_Statistics/NCHS/Publications/ICD10CM/2009/.

American Psychiatric Association. *Diagnostic and Statistical Manual of Mental Disorders.* 4th ed. Washington, DC: the American Psychiatric Association; 2004.

End-of-Chapter Questions

1   The *ICD-10-CM Official Guidelines for Coding and Reporting* are organized into which sections?

    _____

    _____

    _____

2   Coding for signs or symptoms should be used only when:

    _____.

3   Laterality is indicated by the _____ character of the code.

4   When an encounter is for a pathological fracture due to a malignancy, what subcategory would the user reference for the diagnosis?

    _____

5   The subcategories for chemotherapy and radiation therapy are:

    _____ and _____.

CHAPTER 7

ICD-10-CM: Chapter-Specific Guidelines for Chapters 7 to 18

OBJECTIVES

- Understand the guidelines for Chapters 7 to 18 in the International Classification of Diseases, Tenth Revision, Clinical Modification (ICD-10-CM)
- Review examples of ICD-10-CM codes relative to the guidelines
- Review comparisons between ICD-9-CM and ICD-10-CM

Introduction

This chapter will cover chapter-specific guidelines in ICD-10-CM for the following:

- Chapter 7 – Diseases of the eye and adnexa
- Chapter 8 – Diseases of the ear and mastoid process
- Chapter 9 – Diseases of the circulatory system
- Chapter 10 – Diseases of the respiratory system
- Chapter 11 – Diseases of the digestive system
- Chapter 12 – Diseases of the skin and subcutaneous tissue
- Chapter 13 – Diseases of the musculoskeletal system and connective tissue
- Chapter 14 – Diseases of the genitourinary system
- Chapter 15 – Pregnancy, childbirth, and the puerperium
- Chapter 16 – Certain conditions originating in the newborn (perinatal period)
- Chapter 17 – Congenital malformations, deformations, and chromosomal abnormalities
- Chapter 18 – Symptoms, signs, and abnormal clinical and laboratory findings, not elsewhere classified.

Chapter-Specific Guidelines

Chapter 7 – Diseases of the Eye and Adnexa

Codes for diseases of the eye and adnexa are located in Chapter 7 of ICD-10-CM. In ICD-9-CM, codes for the eye and adnexa are reported in the nervous system category. In ICD-10-CM, this category has its own chapter. For most of the categories in Chapter 7, codes are based on laterality. Most codes in this chapter are selected for right eye, left eye, and bilateral (both eyes). In cases in which a code does not provide a designation for which eye is involved, that condition is always bilateral. In cases where a bilateral is not documented, the condition is always assumed unilateral. If the site (left versus right) is not identified, the condition is reported as unspecified.

This chapter contains the following blocks:

- H00–H05   Disorders of eyelid, lacrimal system, and orbit
- H10–H13   Disorders of conjunctiva
- H15–H21   Disorders of sclera, cornea, iris, and ciliary body
- H25–H28   Disorders of lens
- H30–H36   Disorders of choroid and retina
- H40–H42   Glaucoma
- H43–H44   Disorders of vitreous body and globe
- H46–H47   Disorders of optic nerve and visual pathways
- H49–H52   Disorders of ocular muscles, binocular movement, accommodation, and refraction
- H53–H54   Visual disturbances and blindness
- H55–H57   Other disorders of eye and adnexa
- H59   Intraoperative and postprocedural complications and disorders of eye and adnexa, not elsewhere classified.

This group of blocks excludes injuries of the eye and adnexa, which are coded in categories S01.1 to S05.

ICD-9-CM combines the eye and ear codes within the nervous system and sense organs category, but ICD-10-CM defines eye and ear codes in a separate chapter. There are no specific official chapter guidelines for diseases of the eye and adnexa. The following will review reporting diagnoses for some common conditions.

Figure 7.1 compares ICD-9-CM and ICD-10-CM for the diagnosis of low tension, open-angle glaucoma.

FIGURE 7.1 Comparison Between ICD-9-CM and ICD-10-CM for Coding of Low Tension, Open-Angle Glaucoma

ICD-9-CM	ICD-10-CM
365 Glaucoma	H40–H42 Glaucoma
365.12 Low-tension, open-angle glaucoma	H40.1 Open-angle glaucoma
	H40.12 Low-tension glaucoma
	H40.121 Low-tension glaucoma, right eye
	H40.122 Low-tension glaucoma, left eye
	H40.123 Low-tension glaucoma, bilateral
	H40.129 Low-tension glaucoma, unspecified eye

ICD-10-CM is more specific with identifying the affected eye—right, left, bilateral, or unspecified eye—whereas ICD-9-CM identifies only the low-tension, open-angle glaucoma without identification of the affected eye.

Here is an example of the differences between ICD-9-CM and ICD-10-CM: A patient was involved in an industrial accident and suffered a traumatic cataract of the left eye. After examination, the general ophthalmologist determined possible optic nerve damage in the left eye and sent the patient to a neuro-opthalmologist for further evaluation. The diagnosis documented in the medical record is total traumatic cataract of the left eye. In ICD-9-CM, the coder must choose the appropriate code from the following options:

366.2x   Traumatic cataract
      366.20   Unspecified traumatic cataract
      366.21   Localized traumatic opacities of cataract
      366.22   Total traumatic cataract
      366.23   Partially resolved traumatic cataract

In ICD-10-CM, within category H26, a traumatic cataract is coded to H26.13 with a sixth digit to identify the affected eye, if known:

H26.13x   Total traumatic cataract
      H26.131   Total traumatic cataract, right eye
      H26.132   Total traumatic cataract, left eye
      H26.133   Total traumatic cataract, bilateral
      H26.139   Total traumatic cataract, unspecified eye

Figure 7.2 compares ICD-9-CM with ICD-10-CM for the diagnosis of total traumatic cataract.

FIGURE 7.2 Comparison Between ICD-9-CM and ICD-10-CM for Coding of Total Traumatic Cataract

ICD-9-CM	ICD-10-CM
366.22 Total traumatic cataract	H26.132 Total traumatic cataract, left eye

ICD-10-CM allows for more specificity. Intraoperative and postprocedural ophthalmologic complications are coded in category H59 (Intraoperative and postprocedural complications and disorders of eye and adnexa, not elsewhere classified). Codes for complications of care are located within the body system chapters, with codes specific to the organ and structures of that body system. The complication codes should be sequenced first, followed by the specific complication or symptom, if applicable to the patient's condition.

For example, a patient who had cataract surgery on the right eye two days earlier was experiencing pain in the right eye. Following a slit lamp examination of the affected eye, the physician discovered lens fragments in the right eye and returned the patient to the operating room to remove the fragments.

In addition to the specific complication, a secondary diagnosis is needed to identify the ocular pain in both ICD-9-CM and ICD-10-CM. In ICD-9-CM, the following codes would apply:

998.82   Cataract fragments in eye following surgery

379.91   Pain in or around eye

In ICD-10-CM, the complication is more specific, as it identifies which eye is affected:

H59.02   Cataract (lens) fragments in eye following cataract surgery
        H59.021   Cataract (lens) fragments in eye following cataract surgery, right eye
        H59.022   Cataract (lens) fragments in eye following cataract surgery, left eye
        H59.023   Cataract (lens) fragments in eye following cataract surgery, bilateral
        H59.029   Cataract (lens) fragments in eye following cataract surgery, unspecified eye

The correct complication code will identify the affected eye and is coded as H59.11 for the right eye. In addition, the ocular pain should be coded as a secondary diagnosis.

Review category H57.1 for ocular pain:

H57.1   Ocular pain
        H57.10   Ocular pain, unspecified eye
        H57.11   Ocular pain, right eye
        H57.12   Ocular pain, left eye
        H57.13   Ocular pain, bilateral

H57.8   Other specified disorders of eye and adnexa

> **DOCUMENTATION TIP**
>
> Laterality is important in coding diseases of the eye and adnexa.

The patient encounter in ICD-10-CM would be coded:

H59.021   Cataract (lens) fragments in eye following cataract surgery, right eye

H57.11   Ocular pain, right eye

Chapter 8 – Diseases of the Ear and Mastoid Process

In ICD-9-CM, diseases of the ear are coded in the nervous system category. In ICD-10-CM, codes for diseases of the ear and mastoid process are located in Chapter 8. This chapter contains the following blocks:

H60–H62	Diseases of external ear
H65–H75	Diseases of middle ear and mastoid
H80–H83	Diseases of inner ear
H90–H94	Other disorders of ear
H95	Intraoperative and postprocedural complication and disorders of ear and mastoid process, not elsewhere classified

As with diseases of the eye and adnexa, specific chapter guidelines have not been incorporated in the official ICD-10-CM guidelines for coding and reporting. The following example will review reporting diagnoses for some common conditions: A patient underwent an initial tympanoplasty (69631) without mastoidectomy in an outpatient hospital surgery department for an attic perforation of the tympanic membrane of the right ear. The different ICD-9-CM and ICD-10-CM codes are compared in Figure 7.3.

FIGURE 7.3 Comparison Between ICD-9-CM and ICD-10-CM for Coding of Attic Perforation of Tympanic Membrane

ICD-9-CM		ICD-10-CM		
384.2	Perforation of tympanic membrane	H72	Perforation of tympanic membrane	
	384.20 Unspecified perforation of tympanic membrane		H72.1	Attic perforation of tympanic membrane
	384.21 Central perforation of tympanic membrane			H72.10 Attic perforation of tympanic membrane, unspecified ear
	384.22 Attic perforation of tympanic membrane			H72.11 Attic perforation of tympanic membrane, right ear
	384.23 Other marginal perforation of tympanic membrane			H72.12 Attic perforation of tympanic membrane, left ear
	384.24 Multiple perforations of tympanic membrane			H72.13 Attic perforation of tympanic membrane, bilateral
	384.25 Total perforation of tympanic membrane			

ICD-10-CM is more specific in identifying the ear affected. The example indicates that the procedure was performed on the right ear, which is reported with H72.11 in ICD-10-CM. In ICD-10-CM, reviewing the choices shows that the most appropriate diagnosis code is 384.22 (Attic perforation of the tympanic membrane). ICD-9-CM is not as specific, as it does not identify which ear is affected. See Figure 7.4.

FIGURE 7.4 Comparison Between ICD-9-CM and ICD-10-CM for Coding of Attic Perforation of Tympanic Membrane

ICD-9-CM	ICD-10-CM
384.22 Attic perforation of tympanic membrane	H72.11 Attic perforation of tympanic membrane, right ear

---

Codes for complications of care are located within the body system chapter specific to the organs and structure of that body system. The condition or disease should be sequenced first, followed by a complication code in block H95: Intraoperative and postprocedural complications and disorders of ear and mastoid process, not elsewhere classified.

For example, a patient with a history of mastoidectomy underwent a revision of the mastoidectomy with apicectomy (69605) for cholesteatoma of the left middle ear and mastoid. During the procedure, the patient experienced hemorrhage of the ear and mastoid process.

Figure 7.5 illustrates the comparison between ICD-9-CM and ICD-10-CM.

FIGURE 7.5 Comparison Between ICD-9-CM and ICD-10-CM for Coding of Cholesteatoma of the Mastoid Process

ICD-9-CM	ICD-10-CM
385.3 Cholesteatoma of middle ear and mastoid	H71.2 Cholesteatoma of mastoid
385.30 Unspecified cholesteatoma	H71.20 Cholesteatoma of mastoid, unspecified ear
385.31 Cholesteatoma of attic	H71.21 Cholesteatoma of mastoid, right ear
385.32 Cholesteatoma of middle ear	H71.22 Cholesteatoma of mastoid, left ear
385.33 Cholesteatoma of middle ear and mastoid	H71.23 Cholesteatoma of mastoid, bilateral
385.35 Diffuse cholesteatosis	H71.3 Diffuse cholesteotosis
	H71.9 Unspecified cholesteotosis

In ICD-10-CM, the diagnosis would be reported with code H71.22 (Cholesteatoma of mastoid, left ear) and with ICD-9-CM, 385.33 (Cholesteatoma of middle ear and mastoid). According to the ICD-10-CM guidelines, the complication is also coded.

Review the options for coding intraoperative and postprocedural complications of the ear (H95.2), as shown below:

H95.2   Intraoperative and postprocedural hemorrhage of ear and mastoid process complicating a procedure

Excludes1: intraoperative hemorrhage or hematoma due to accidental puncture or laceration during a procedure on the ear (H95.3-)

H95.21   Intraoperative hematoma of the ear and mastoid process during a procedure of the ear and mastoid process

H95.22   Intraoperative hematoma of other organ or structure during a procedure of the ear and mastoid process

The most appropriate complication code in this block is H95.23 (Intraoperative hematoma of the ear and mastoid process during a procedure of the ear and mastoid process).

DOCUMENTATION TIP

Codes for the ear are based on laterality.

Chapter 9 – Diseases of the Circulatory System

Hypertensive heart disease is coded in Chapter 9 of ICD-10-CM. Codes in this classification are found in categories I10 to I15. There are many differences between ICD-9-CM and ICD-10-CM regarding this classification. Under hypertensive disease, there are instructional notes to use an additional code when the patient has:

- a history of tobacco use (Z87.891);
- exposure to environmental tobacco smoke (Z72.22);
- occupational exposure to environmental tobacco smoke (Z57.31);
- tobacco dependence (F17.-); or
- tobacco use (Z72.0).

This category also excludes hypertensive disease complicating pregnancy, childbirth, and the puerperium; neonatal hypertension; and pulmonary hypertension. Category I10 would be reported when the diagnostic statement indicates the hypertension is under control or uncontrolled with therapy. Elevated blood pressure without further specificity is not coded in this category but is assigned to R03.0. Code R03.0 may also be used for a single elevated blood pressure reading or for transient elevated blood pressure.

For example, a patient who had been treated for hypertension for more than three years visited his internist for a 3-month follow-up. He smoked currently but was not dependent on tobacco. His blood pressure was 150/100 mm Hg. The physician adjusted the dose of the patient's medication, reviewed previous blood pressure readings, counseled the patient regarding smoking cessation, and asked the patient to come back in two months. The documentation indicates benign hypertension without good control.

The comparison between ICD-9-CM and ICD-10-CM is shown in Figure 7.6.

FIGURE 7.6 **Comparison Between ICD-9-CM and ICD-10-CM for Coding of Essential Hypertension**

ICD-9-CM			ICD-10-CM	
401	Essential hypertension		I10	Essential (primary) hypertension
	401.0	Essential hypertension, malignant		Includes: high blood pressure
				benign
	401.1	Essential hypertension, benign		arterial
				essential
	401.9	Unspecified essential hypertension		malignant
				primary
				systemic in this category

In ICD-9-CM, the correct code is 401.1 (Essential hypertension, benign). In ICD-10-CM, the correct codes are I10 (Essential (primary) hypertension) and Z72.0 (Tobacco use). Remember, with category I10, an additional code is reported for tobacco exposure, dependence, or use. This differs from coding in ICD-9-CM. There is an *Excludes2* note indicating that hypertension (I10) may be reported in addition to the following:

Essential (primary) hypertension involving vessels of brain (I60-I69)
Essential (primary) hypertension involving vessels of eye (H35.0).

Category H35.0 is reported for hypertensive retinopathy and may be used alone or with I10. If both codes are used, the sequencing is based on the reason for the encounter.

For example, a patient presented to the ophthalmologist for follow-up of hypertensive retinopathy. The physician determined that the retinopathy was a result of the patient's malignant hypertension. See Figure 7.7.

FIGURE 7.7 **Comparison Between ICD-9-CM and ICD-10-CM for Coding of Hypertensive Retinopathy**

ICD-9-CM		ICD-10-CM	
362.11	Hypertensive retinopathy	H35.033	Hypertensive retinopathy, bilateral
		I10	Essential (primary) hypertension

In ICD-9-CM, the hypertension is not reported. There is an instruction note with 401.x that excludes hypertension with the eye (362.11). The *Excludes2* note allows reporting of both codes in ICD-10-CM.

Hypertensive Heart Disease

Hypertensive heart disease is classifed in category I11. Hypertensive heart disease diagnoses are combination codes that include both the hypertension and the heart disease. There is an *includes* note that indicates what conditions are included with hypertension in category I11. A causal relationship does not need to be documented. For hypertension with heart failure, a secondary code is required from category I50- to identify the type of heart failure.

Review category I11 for hypertensive heart disease.

I11   Hypertensive heart disease
              Includes: any condition in I51.4-I51.9 due to hypertension

        I11.0   Hypertensive heart disease with heart failure
                    Hypertensive heart failure
                    Use additional code to identify type of heart failure (I50.-)

        I11.9   Hypertensive heart disease without heart failure
                    Hypertensive heart disease NOS

For example, an established patient was treated by a cardiologist for hypertensive heart disease with benign hypertension. The patient was doing well, and after completing a detailed history and examination, the physician determined that the current regimen was effective and that she would see the patient in six weeks. Figure 7.8 illustrates the differences between ICD-9-CM and ICD-10-CM for coding in this situation.

FIGURE 7.8 **Comparison Between ICD-9-CM and ICD-10-CM for Coding of Hypertensive Heart Disease Without Failure**

ICD-9-CM		ICD-10-CM	
402.10	Benign hypertensive heart disease	I11.9	Hypertensive heart disease without heart failure

---

Because the practitioner did not identify heart failure in the documentation, only one code is reported for ICD-9-CM and ICD-10-CM.

Hypertensive Chronic Kidney Disease

In ICD-9-CM, the term *renal disease* was replaced with *chronic kidney disease*. The same is true in ICD-10-CM. Hypertensive chronic kidney disease codes are combination codes that include both hypertension and chronic kidney disease and are coded in category I12. There is an *includes* note specifying what conditions are included in this category. If a patient has both a condition listed in the *includes* note and hypertension, the combination code category I12 is reported, not individual codes for hypertensive chronic kidney disease. If a patient has hypertension with both chronic kidney disease and acute renal failure, an additional code (category N18) for the acute renal failure is required. See Figures 7.9 and 7.10.

**FIGURE 7.9 Excerpt From ICD-10-CM I12
Hypertensive Chronic Kidney Disease**

I12 **Hypertensive chronic kidney disease**

Includes: any condition in N18.- due to any condition in I10

arteriosclerosis of kidney

arteriosclerotic nephritis (chronic) (interstitial)

hypertensive nephropathy

nephrosclerosis

Excludes1: hypertension due to kidney disease (I15.0, I15.1)

renovascular hypertension (I15.0)

secondary hypertension (I15.-)

Excludes2: acute renal failure (N17.-)

I12.0 Hypertensive chronic kidney disease with stage V chronic kidney disease or end-stage renal disease

Use additional code to identify the stage of chronic kidney disease (N18.5, N18.6)

I12.9 Hypertensive chronic kidney disease with stage I through stage IV chronic kidney disease, or unspecified chronic kidney disease

Hypertensive chronic kidney disease NOS

Hypertensive renal disease NOS

Use additional code to identify the stage of chronic kidney disease (N18.1, N18.4, N18.9)

**FIGURE 7.10 Excerpt From ICD-10-CM
Tabular List, N18**

N18 **Chronic kidney disease (CKD)**

Code first any associated: diabetic chronic kidney disease (E08.22, E09.22, E10.22, E11.22, E13.22), hypertensive chronic kidney disease (I12.-, I13.-)

Use additional code to identify kidney transplant status, if applicable, (Z94.0)

N18.1 Chronic kidney disease, stage I

N18.2 Chronic kidney disease, stage II (mild)

N18.3 Chronic kidney disease, stage III (moderate)

N18.4 Chronic kidney disease, stage IV (severe)

N18.5 Chronic kidney disease, stage V

Excludes1: chronic kidney disease, stage V requiring chronic dialysis (N18.6)

N18.6 End-stage renal disease

Chronic kidney disease requiring chronic dialysis

Use additional code to identify dialysis status (Z99.2)

N18.9 Chronic kidney disease, unspecified

Chronic renal disease

Chronic renal failure NOS

Chronic renal insufficiency

Chronic uremia

For example, a patient with malignant hypertension and stage V chronic renal disease was admitted to the critical care unit. The patient was in acute renal failure with acute cortical necrosis. Two codes are reported in ICD-9-CM and in ICD-10-CM. A code is selected for the hypertensive chronic kidney disease along with the stage of the chronic kidney disease. Figure 7.11 illustrates the comparison between ICD-9-CM and ICD-10-CM.

FIGURE 7.11 Comparison Between ICD-9-CM and ICD-10-CM for Coding of Hypertensive Chronic Kidney Disease

ICD-9-CM		ICD-10-CM	
403.01	Hypertensive chronic kidney disease, malignant	I12.0	Hypertensive chronic kidney disease with stage V chronic kidney disease or end-stage renal disease
585.5	Chronic kidney disease, stage V	N18.5	Chronic kidney disease, stage V

GUIDELINE TIP

Remember to code the acute renal failure when the patient is diagnosed with both acute and chronic renal failure.

Hypertensive Heart and Chronic Kidney Disease

Hypertensive heart and chronic kidney disease codes that are combination codes, which include hypertension, heart disease, and kidney disease, are coded in category I13.

The *includes* note in category I13 specifies that the conditions in I11 and I13 are included. If the patient has hypertension, heart disease, and chronic kidney disease, a code from this category is reported. In addition, for patients with heart failure, a code from category I50 is reported as an additional code.

If the patient is diagnosed with both acute and chronic renal failure, a code from category N17 or N19 is required for the acute renal failure.

The guidelines in ICD-9-CM and ICD-10-CM both have an additional instructional note to use an additional code to identify the stage of chronic kidney disease. Both ICD-9-CM and ICD-10-CM require an additional code for reporting the type of heart failure. See Figure 7.12.

FIGURE 7.12 **Comparison Between ICD-9-CM and ICD-10-CM for Coding of Hypertensive Heart and Chronic Kidney Disease**

ICD-9-CM	ICD-10-CM
404.9 **Hypertensive heart and chronic kidney disease, unspecified**	**I13** **Hypertensive heart and chronic kidney disease**
404.90 Hypertensive heart and chronic kidney disease, unspecified, without heart failure and with chronic kidney disease stage I through stage IV, or unspecified	Includes: any condition in I11.- with any condition in I12.- cardiorenal disease cardiovascular renal disease
404.91 Hypertensive heart and chronic kidney disease, unspecified, with heart failure and with chronic kidney disease stage I through stage IV, or unspecified	**I13.2** **Hypertensive heart and chronic kidney disease with heart failure and with stage V chronic kidney disease, or end-stage renal disease**
404.92 Hypertensive heart and chronic kidney disease, unspecified, without heart failure and with chronic kidney disease stage V or end-stage renal disease	Use additional code to identify type of heart failure (I50.-) Use additional code to identify the stage of chronic kidney disease (N18.5, N18.6)
404.93 Hypertensive heart and chronic kidney disease, unspecified, with heart failure and chronic kidney disease stage V or end-stage renal disease	

For example, a patient was admitted to the hospital with acute diastolic heart failure due to hypertension with end-stage renal disease. Review the comparison between ICD-9-CM and ICD-10-CM in Figure 7.13.

FIGURE 7.13 **Comparison Between ICD-9-CM and ICD-10-CM for Coding of Hypertensive Heart and Chronic Kidney Disease**

ICD-9-CM		ICD-10-CM	
404.91	Hypertensive heart and chronic kidney disease, unspecified, with heart failure and with chronic kidney disease stage I through stage IV, or unspecified	I13.2	Hypertensive heart and renal disease with both heart failure and chronic renal failure
428.0	Congestive heart failure, unspecified	I50.31	Acute diastolic (congestive) heart failure
585.6	End-stage renal disease	N18.6	End-stage renal disease

Because the guidelines specify reporting of both the acute heart failure and the end-stage renal disease in addition to the hypertensive heart and chronic kidney disease, all three codes would be reported for both ICD-9-CM and ICD-10-CM.

Secondary Hypertension

Secondary hypertension is due to an underlying condition. Secondary hypertension is not coded in a manifestation category. Two codes are required when coding from category I15—one to identify the underlying etiology and one from I15 to identify the hypertension. Sequencing of the codes is based on the reason for the encounter.

There are two *excludes* notes: Excludes1: postoperative hypertension (I97.3); Excludes2: secondary hypertension involving vessels of brain (I60-I69) and secondary hypertension involving vessels of eye (H35.0).

Remember that when there is an *Excludes 1* note, the code that is excluded may not be used in addition to the code from category I15 for secondary hypertension. The *Excludes 2* note allows reporting I15 (secondary hypertension) with the condition.

I15   Secondary Hypertension
   Code also underlying condition
   Excludes1: postoperative hypertension (I97.3)
   Excludes2: secondary hypertension involving vessels of
      brain (I60-I69)
   secondary hypertension involving vessels of eye (H35.0) I15.0

   I15.0   Renovascular hypertension
   I15.1   Hypertension secondary to other renal disorders
   I15.2   Hypertension secondary to endocrine disorders
   I15.8   Other secondary hypertension
   I15.9   Secondary hypertension, unspecified

In ICD-9-CM, secondary hypertension is reported with one code from category 405.5x to identify what the secondary hypertension results from. The x represent a fourth and fifth digit to report whether the secondary hypertension is malignant, benign, or unspecified. One exception is secondary hypertension due to glomerulosclerosis, which is coded as 403.5.

For example, a patient was treated for malignant renal occlusion secondary to hypertension. Figure 7.14 illustrates the comparison between ICD-9-CM and ICD-10-CM codes in this situation.

> **GUIDELINES TIP**
>
> Remember that when there is an *Excludes 1* note, the code that is excluded may not be used.

FIGURE 7.14 Comparison Between ICD-9-CM and ICD-10-CM for Coding of Secondary Hypertension

ICD-9-CM		ICD-10-CM	
405.09	Other secondary hypertension	I15.0	Renovascular hypertension
593.81	Vascular disorders of kidney	N28.0	Ischemia and infarction of kidney
	Renal (artery):		Malignant renal artery occlusion
	embolism		
	hemorrhage		
	thrombosis		
	Renal infarction		

In ICD-9-CM, two codes are required—one to identify the underlying etiology and one to identify the hypertension in category 405. In ICD-10-CM, a combination code does not exist, and the renal artery occlusion must be reported as well as the renovascular hypertension, based on ICD-10-CM draft guidelines.

Hypertension Controlled

The term *hypertension controlled* generally refers to a patient whose hypertension is under control. In ICD-10-CM, the code assignment is I10.

Hypertension Uncontrolled

Hypertension uncontrolled is defined as hypertension either untreated or not responding to the current therapeutic regimen. It should be coded using I10 for hypertension, regardless of whether the hypertension is controlled or uncontrolled. Figure 7.15 illustrates coding for *hypertension controlled* in ICD-10-CM.

FIGURE 7.15 **Excerpt From ICD-10-CM Tabular List, I10**

I10   Essential (primary) hypertension

Includes: high blood pressure, hypertension (arterial) (benign) (essential) (malignant) (primary) (systemic)

Excludes1: hypertensive disease complicating pregnancy, childbirth, and the puerperium (O10-O11, O13-O16)

Excludes2: essential (primary) hypertension involving vessels of brain (I60-I69), essential (primary) hypertension involving vessels of eye (H35.0)

In ICD-9-CM, hypertension is reported with three codes classified in category 401.

401   Essential hypertension
    401.0   Malignant hypertension
    401.1   Benign
    401.9   Unspecified

In ICD-10-CM, category I10 includes malignant, benign, and unspecified hypertension with one code. In ICD-9-CM, elevated blood pressure is without further specificity and is coded as 796.2 (Elevated blood pressure). In ICD-10-CM, elevated blood pressure is coded as R03.0 and is reported for an elevated blood pressure reading or for transient elevated blood pressure. See Figure 7.16.

FIGURE 7.16 **Comparison Between ICD-9-CM and ICD-10-CM for Coding of Elevated Blood Pressure**

ICD-9-CM	ICD-10-CM
796.2 Elevated blood pressure reading without diagnosis of hypertension	R03.0 Elevated blood pressure reading, without diagnosis of hypertension

Atherosclerotic Coronary Artery Disease and Angina

Combination codes are used for atherosclerotic heart disease with angina pectoris. Two codes are used—I25.110-125.119 (Atherosclerotic heart disease of native coronary artery with angina pectoris) and I25.709 (Atherosclerosis of coronary artery bypass graft[s] and coronary artery of transplanted heart with angina pectoris). The codes identify the type of angina.

For example, a patient with unstable angina with coronary artery atherosclerosis was admitted to the hospital for treatment. Review the comparison between ICD-9-CM and ICD-10-CM in Figure 7.17.

FIGURE 7.17 Comparison Between ICD-9-CM and ICD-10-CM for Coding of Atherosclerotic Heart Disease

ICD-9-CM		ICD-10-CM	
414.01	Coronary atherosclerosis of native coronary artery	I25.110	Atherosclerotic heart disease of native coronary artery with
413.9	Angina (pectoris)		unstable angina pectoris

ICD-10-CM uses only one combination code to report this condition. When a combination code is used, it is not necessary to report an additional code for the angina, unless the documentation indicates that the angina is due to a condition other than atherosclerosis. The angina does not have to be documented to a specified occluded artery. When a patient is admitted because of an acute myocardial infarction, the myocardial infarction is sequenced before the coronary artery disease.

Initial and subsequent myocardial infarction in ICD-10-CM has two categories:

I21   Acute myocardial infarction

I22   Subsequent myocardial infarction.

I21 is reported for all cases of initial myocardial infarction. This code is to be used from the onset of the myocardial infarction until four weeks following onset. Code I22 is reported when a patient suffers an acute myocardial infarction and has a new onset within the four-week time frame of the initial myocardial infarction. A code from I22 may be used in conjunction with category I21, and sequencing depends on the circumstance of the encounter.

Circumstance 1

If a patient has an acute myocardial infarction and is admitted to the hospital and while still in the hospital suffers another acute myocardial infarction, category I21 would be sequenced first, followed by category I22 as a secondary code.

For example, a patient was admitted to the critical care unit from the emergency department after suffering an acute myocardial infarction of the left main coronary artery. Two days later, the patient suffered a second myocardial infarction (acute) of the inferior wall. The correct code reporting would be as follows:

Principal/first listed diagnosis code:

> I21.01   ST elevation (STEMI) myocardial infarction involving left main coronary artery

Secondary diagnosis code:

> I22.1   Subsequent ST elevation (STEMI) myocardial infarction of inferior wall

Circumstance 2

When a patient has a subsequent acute myocardial infarction after discharge after the initial myocardial infarction, and the reason for the admission is the second or subsequent acute myocardial infarction, category I22 is sequenced first, followed by a secondary code from category I21. The I21 code indicates the site of the initial acute myocardial infarction and indicates that the patient is still within the four-week time frame of healing from the initial acute myocardial infarction. Review code category I21 for acute myocardial infarction of the anterior wall. Review Figures 7.18 and 7.19 with the following example: A patient was admitted to the hospital suffering from an acute myocardial infarction of the inferior wall. The patient was released three weeks earlier after suffering an acute myocardial infarction of the left anterior descending coronary artery. The correct code reporting is as follows:

> Principal/first listed diagnosis code–I22.1 Subsequent ST elevation (STEMI) myocardial infarction of inferior wall
> Secondary diagnosis code–I21.02 ST elevation (STEMI) myocardial infarction involving left anterior descending coronary artery.

FIGURE 7.18 **Excerpt From ICD-10-CM, Category I21**

I21   ST elevation (STEMI) and non-ST elevation (NSTEMI) myocardial infarction
          Includes: cardiac infarction
     I21.0   ST elevation (STEMI) myocardial infarction of anterior wall
          I21.01   ST elevation (STEMI) myocardial infarction involving
                          left main coronary artery
          I21.02   ST elevation (STEMI) myocardial infarction involving
                          left anterior descending coronary artery
                     ST elevation (STEMI) myocardial infarction involving diagonal
                          coronary artery
          I21.09   ST elevation (STEMI) myocardial infarction involving other
                          coronary artery of anterior wall
                     Acute transmural myocardial infarction of anterior wall
                     Anteroapical transmural (Q wave) infarction (acute)
                     Anterolateral transmural (Q wave) infarction (acute)
                     Anteroseptal transmural (Q wave) infarction (acute)
                     Transmural (Q wave) infarction (acute) (of) anterior
                          (wall) NOS

> **FIGURE 7.19 Excerpt From ICD-10-CM, Category I22**
>
> I22.1   Subsequent ST elevation (STEMI) myocardial infarction of inferior wall
>   Subsequent acute transmural myocardial infarction of inferior wall
>   Subsequent transmural (Q wave) infarction (acute)(of) diaphragmatic wall
>   Subsequent transmural (Q wave) infarction (acute)(of) inferior (wall) NOS
>   Subsequent inferolateral transmural (Q wave) infarction (acute)
>   Subsequent inferoposterior transmural (Q wave) infarction (acute)

When both acute myocardial infarction and atherosclerotic coronary artery disease are documented in the medical record, the acute myocardial infarction is sequenced first, followed by the coronary artery disease code. Cardiac arrest is coded as follows:

I46   Cardiac arrest
           Excludes1: cardiogenic shock (R57.0)

    I46.2   Cardiac arrest due to underlying cardiac condition
                   Code first underlying cardiac condition

    I46.8   Cardiac arrest due to other underlying condition
                   Code first underlying condition

    I46.9   Cardiac arrest, cause unspecified.

Cardiac arrest, cause unspecified, is acceptable as the principal diagnosis only if the patient expires or is discharged within 24 hours of admission to the hospital or emergency department and a cause of cardiac arrest cannot be determined. Do not use I46.9 as a secondary diagnosis unless the cause is not documented.

If a patient goes into cardiac arrest while being treated for an underlying cardiac condition (I46.8), the cardiac arrest is coded as the secondary diagnosis. Codes in category I46 should not be used as the principal diagnosis when an underlying cause is known.

For example, during a recent hospitalization, a patient treated for congestive cardiomyopathy went into cardiac arrest. The patient was revived and transferred to the coronary care unit after stabilization.

ICD-10-CM: Principal/first listed diagnosis–I42.0 Dilated cardiomyopathy
                    (congestive cardiomyopathy)
Secondary diagnosis–I46.2 Cardiac arrest due to underlying cardiac condition

GUIDELINE TIP

If an attempt to resuscitate a patient who suffers a cardiac arrest is not successful, the encounter is still coded.

There are three categories in ICD-10-CM for coding occlusion and stenosis of the precerebral and cerebral arteries either with or without the presence of cerebral infarction. The three categories are as follows:

I63   Cerebral infarction

I65   Occlusion and stenosis of precerebral arteries, not resulting in cerebral infarction

I66   Occlusion and stenosis of cerebral arteries, not resulting in cerebral infarction

Category I63 identifies the cerebral infarction at the fourth character level and identifies the site and type of infarction. Category I66 is for use when there is evidence of obstruction of a vessel without evidence of infarct. A cerebrovascular accident, not specified, is coded as I63.9 (Cerebral infarction, unspecified stroke NOS). A code from category I69 is reported when a complication of an intracerebral hemorrhage or infarction is documented and may be used after the initial CVA. The term *sequelae* is defined as "the after-effect of a disease, condition, or injury, or a secondary result" (www.merriam-webster .com/dictionary/sequelae).This category has a six-character extension. Review Figure 7.20.

FIGURE 7.20 **Excerpt from ICD-10-CM Tabular List, I69**

I69   **Sequelae of cerebrovascular disease**

       Note: This category is to be used to indicate conditions in I60-I67 as the cause of sequelae. The sequelae include conditions specified as such or as residuals, which may occur at any time after the onset of the causal condition.

       Excludes1: personal history of cerebral infarction without
             residual deficit (Z86.73),
             personal history of prolonged reversible ischemic
             neurologic deficit (PRIND) (Z86.73),
             personal history of reversible ischemic neurological
             deficit (RIND) (Z86.73),
             sequelae of traumatic intracranial injury (S06.-),
             transient ischemic attack (TIA) (G45.9)

If a patient has a personal history of a transient ischemic attack and cerebral infarction without any documented residual deficits, use Z86.73 as an additional diagnosis for a patient with a history of cerebrovascular disease when no neurologic defects are present.

Chapter 10 – Diseases of the Respiratory System

Chronic obstructive pulmonary disease (COPD) is coded as J44 (Other chronic obstructive pulmonary disease). Conditions in this category include the following:

- Asthma with chronic obstructive pulmonary disease
- Chronic asthmatic (obstructive) bronchitis
- Chronic bronchitis with airway obstruction

- Chronic bronchitis with emphysema
- Chronic emphysematous bronchitis
- Chronic obstructive asthma
- Chronic obstructive bronchitis
- Chronic obstructive tracheobronchitis.

Diagnosis codes J44- and J45- distinguish between uncomplicated cases of chronic obstructive bronchitis and asthma and those that are in acute exacerbation. J44- is used to report chronic obstructive pulmonary disease, and J45- is for reporting asthma. See Figure 7.21.

FIGURE 7.21 Excerpt From ICD-10-CM Tabular List, J44.0

J44.0   Chronic obstructive pulmonary disease with acute lower
         respiratory infection
              Use additional code to identify the infection

J44.1   Chronic obstructive pulmonary disease with (acute) exacerbation
              Decompensated COPD
              Decompensated COPD with (acute) exacerbation
              Excludes2: chronic obstructive pulmonary disease [COPD] with
                  acute bronchitis (J44.0)

J44.9   Chronic obstructive pulmonary disease, unspecified
              Chronic obstructive airway disease NOS
              Chronic obstructive lung disease NOS

Any combination not included in J44- is reported separately. For example, the codes in category J44 indicate whether the patient has an uncomplicated case, an acute exacerbation, or a coexisting lower respiratory tract infection. The code for the lower respiratory tract infection takes precedence over the acute exacerbation. If the infection is pneumonia or influenza, a secondary code for the type of pneumonia or influenza is required.

For example, a patient with COPD was admitted by her internist with a diagnosis of COPD with respiratory syncytial virus pneumonia. The encounter is reported with the following codes in ICD-10-CM:

Principal/first listed diagnosis–J44.0	Chronic obstructive pulmonary disease with acute lower respiratory Infection
Secondary diagnosis–J12.1	Respiratory syncytial virus pneumonia

Nosocomial Respiratory Infections

If a patient contracts a respiratory infection while in the hospital, a code from Y95 is assigned along with a code for the type of infection. The infection is reported as the principal/first listed diagnosis.

For example, a hospitalized patient developed a staphylococcal infection and was treated with antibiotics. The encounter is reported as follows:

Principal/first listed diagnosis–B95.8	Unspecified staphylococcus as the cause of diseases classified elsewhere
Secondary diagnosis–Y95	Nosocomial condition

GUIDELINE TIP

Remember to code the underlying condition when reporting cardiac arrest, if applicable.

Avian Influenza

Only confirmed cases of avian influenza should be reported. Coding is based on the provider's medical record documentation to support reporting this condition, which is reported with subcategory J09. Confirmation based on positive laboratory serology test results is not required. If the provider suspects or documents *probable* avian influenza, a code from category J10 (Influenza due to other influenza virus) is used.

For example, a patient was treated in the emergency department with influenza-like symptoms. The patient had recently returned from a trip to Hong Kong and was exposed to avian influenza virus. The physician documented in the medical record, "influenza, suspect probably avian influenza." The correct code reported is J10.1 (Influenza NOS).

Chapter 11 – Diseases of the Digestive System

Ulcers are coded using the following categories:
- K25   Gastric ulcer
- K26   Duodenal ulcer
- K27   Peptic ulcer
- K28   Gastrojejunal ulcer.

These codes are combination codes that identify complications of ulcers (bleeding and perforation). A secondary code is not required unless the patient had multiple complications.

Currently there are no specific chapter guidelines for diseases of the digestive system. This section is a review of some conditions found in this chapter of ICD-10-CM. Review Figure 7.22.

FIGURE 7.22 Excerpt From ICD-10-CM Tabular List, K25

K25   Gastric ulcer

Includes: erosion (acute) of stomach, pylorus ulcer (peptic), stomach ulcer (peptic)

Use additional code to identify:

alcohol abuse and dependence (F10.-)

Excludes1: acute gastritis (K29.0-), peptic ulcer NOS (K27.-)

K25.0   Acute gastric ulcer with hemorrhage

K25.1   Acute gastric ulcer with perforation

K25.2   Acute gastric ulcer with both hemorrhage and perforation

K25.3   Acute gastric ulcer without hemorrhage or perforation

K25.4   Chronic or unspecified gastric ulcer with hemorrhage

K25.5   Chronic or unspecified gastric ulcer with perforation

K25.6   Chronic or unspecified gastric ulcer with both hemorrhage and perforation

K25.7   Chronic gastric ulcer without hemorrhage or perforation

K25.9   Gastric ulcer, unspecified as acute or chronic, without hemorrhage or perforation

---

For example, a patient was admitted by his family physician with an acute gastric ulcer that had perforated. Review the coding comparison between ICD-9-CM and ICD-10-CM in Figure 7.23.

FIGURE 7.23 Comparison Between ICD-9-CM and ICD-10-CM for Coding of Acute Gastric Ulcer

ICD-9-CM		ICD-10-CM	
531.10	Gastric ulcer, acute with perforation without mention of obstruction	K25.1	Acute gastric ulcer with perforation

---

Notice that a combination code also exists with ICD-9-CM. Crohn's disease is classified in category K50 in ICD-10-CM. Codes in this category have much more detail than in ICD-9-CM. Review the codes in category K50.

K50.9   Crohn's disease, unspecified

K50.90   Crohn's disease, unspecified, without complications

Crohn's disease NOS

Regional enteritis NOS

K50.91   Crohn's disease, unspecified, with complications

K50.911   Crohn's disease, unspecified, with rectal bleeding

K50.912   Crohn's disease, unspecified, with intestinal obstruction

K50.913   Crohn's disease, unspecified, with fistula

> K50.914   Crohn's disease, unspecified, with abscess
> K50.918   Crohn's disease, unspecified, with other complication
> K50.919   Crohn's disease, unspecified, with unspecified complications

If a patient has multiple complications, multiple codes may be reported from K50 or K51 (ulcerative colitis) to report each complication. Review the comparison in ICD-9-CM. Crohn's disease is classified in category 555 (regional enteritis).

555.4   Regional enteritis
>   Includes: Crohn's disease
>   Granulomatous enteritis

555.0   Small intestine

555.1   Large intestine

555.2   Small intestine with large intestine

555.9   Unspecified site
>   Crohn's disease NOS
>   Regional enteritis (NOS)

For example, a patient was diagnosed with Crohn's disease complicated by rectal bleeding. Review the comparison between ICD-9-CM and ICD-10-CM as shown in Figure 7.24. In ICD-9-CM, there is no combination code for Crohn's disease with rectal bleeding, and both codes must be reported separately. In ICD-10-CM, there is a combination code for the condition, so only one code is required.

FIGURE 7.24 **Comparison Between ICD-9-CM and ICD-10-CM for Coding of Crohn's Disease With Rectal Bleeding**

ICD-9-CM		ICD-10-CM	
555.9	Crohn's disease, unspecified site	K50.911	Crohn's disease, unspecified, with rectal bleeding
569.3	Hemorrhage of rectum or anus (rectal bleeding)		

GUIDELINE TIP

Secondary codes are not required when ulcers are coded unless the patient has multiple complications.

Chapter 12 – Diseases of the Skin and Subcutaneous Tissue

In 2010, guidelines were added for Diseases of Skin and Subcutaneous Tissue in relation to pressure ulcers. This section is a review of some conditions found in this chapter of ICD-10-CM.

Pressure Ulcers

Pressure ulcer stages. Codes from category L89, Pressure ulcer, are combination codes that identify the site of the pressure ulcer as well as the stage of the ulcer.

The ICD-10-CM classifies pressure ulcer stages based on severity, which is designated by stages 1-4, unspecified stage and unstageable. Assign as many codes from category L89 as needed to identify all the pressure ulcers the patient has, if applicable.

Unstageable pressure ulcers

Assignment of the code for unstageable pressure ulcer (L89.—) should be based on the clinical documentation. These codes are used for pressure ulcers, whose stage cannot be clinically determined (eg, the ulcer is covered by eschar or has been treated with a skin or muscle graft) and pressure ulcers that are documented as deep tissue injury but not documented as due to trauma. This code should not be confused with the codes for unspecified stage (L89.—). When there is no documentation regarding the stage of the pressure ulcer, assign the appropriate code for unspecified stage (L89.—).

Documented pressure ulcer stage

Assignment of the pressure ulcer stage code should be guided by clinical documentation of the stage or documentation of the terms found in the index. For clinical terms describing the stage that are not found in the index, and there is no documentation of the stage, the provider should be queried. A code from this category is not assigned if the documentation states the pressure ulcer is completely healed.

Patients admitted with pressure ulcers documented as healing

Pressure ulcers described as healing should be assigned the appropriate pressure ulcer stage code based on the documentation in the medical record. If the documentation does not provide information about the stage of the healing pressure ulcer, assign the appropriate code for unspecified stage.

If the documentation is unclear as to whether the patient has a current (new) pressure ulcer or if the patient is being treated for a healing pressure ulcer, query the provider.

Patient admitted with pressure ulcer evolving into another stage during the admission

If a patient is admitted with a pressure ulcer at one stage and it progresses to a higher stage, assign the code for the highest stage reported for that site.

Documentation for BMI and Pressure Ulcer Stages

For the Body Mass Index (BMI) and pressure ulcer stage codes, code assignment may be based on medical record documentation from clinicians who are not the patient's provider (i.e., physician or other qualified healthcare practitioner legally accountable for establishing the patient's diagnosis), since this information is typically documented by other clinicians involved in the care of the patient (eg, a dietitian often documents the BMI and nurses often documents the pressure ulcer stages). However, the associated diagnosis (such as overweight, obesity, or pressure ulcer) must be documented by the patient's provider. If there is conflicting medical record documentation, either from the same clinician or different clinicians, the patient's attending provider should be queried for clarification.

The BMI codes should only be reported as secondary diagnoses with Z68.-. As with all other secondary diagnosis codes, the BMI codes should only be assigned when they meet the definition of a reportable additional diagnosis.

Codes for decubitus ulcers are classified in L89 and nondecubitus ulcers in L97. Both are coded with a sixth character extension. The fifth character identifies the site of the ulcer, and the sixth character is used for reporting the depth of the ulcer. If gangrene is present, it is reported first as I96. Decubitus ulcers in this category include the following:

- Bed sores
- Plaster ulcer
- Pressure area
- Pressure sore.

Nondecubitus ulcers include the following:

- Chronic ulcer of the skin
- Nonhealing ulcer of skin
- Noninfected sinus of skin
- Trophic ulcer NOS
- Tropical ulcer NOS
- Ulcer of skin NOS.

For coding of decubitus and nondecubitus ulcers, the site and depth must be documented in the medical record. When multiple ulcers are documented in the medical record, only the most severe ulcer of the same site is coded. Decubitus ulcers may occur at multiple sites. A decubitus ulcer that has become serious and does not respond to treatment may support medical necessity for hospital admission. If the reason for admission is the decubitus ulcer, it should be reported as the principal/first listed diagnosis. Secondary codes for other problems or problems associated with the decubitus ulcer should be reported also.

If the patient has an underlying condition, such as diabetes mellitus or atherosclerosis of the lower extremities, it should be coded as the first listed diagnosis followed by the code for the nondecubitus ulcer. The codes for diabetes mellitus and atherosclerosis do include the extremity ulcers, but L97- will identify the site and depth of the ulcer and should also be reported.

It is common with these conditions for patients to develop these types of ulcers. If there is no underlying cause or condition, the nondecubitus ulcer is listed first. There is an instructional note for both of these categories to code first gangrene if present. Review the following example: A patient with type 2 diabetes was treated in a wound care center in an outpatient hospital department for a chronic, nondecubitus foot ulcer of the heel and midfoot. The physician diagnosed the condition as necrotizing to the bone. The encounter is coded using ICD-10-CM as follows:

Principal/first listed diagnosis–E11.621	Type 2 diabetes mellitus with foot ulcer
Secondary diagnosis–L97.404	Nonpressure chronic ulcer of unspecified heel and midfoot with necrosis of bone

Code L56.0 and L56.1 describe phototoxic and photoallergic responses or changes due to ultraviolet radiation. These codes identify a dermatologic condition due to a drug or chemical. Codes from poisoning and adverse effects of drugs, medicaments, and biological substances (T51–T65) or a code to identify the drug or chemical (T36–T50) are reported as the first listed diagnosis, followed by a code from L56.0- and L56.1-.

Category L57 is reported for skin changes due to chronic exposure to nonionizing radiation. A secondary external cause (W89, X32) code is reported to identify the source of the exposure.

For example, a patient had a photoallergic response from an adverse effect of penicillin. The patient was seeing a dermatologist for treatment.

Principal/first listed diagnosis–T36.0x5	Adverse effect of penicillins
Secondary diagnosis–L56.1	Drug photoallergic response

Chapter 13 – Diseases of the Musculoskeletal System and Connective Tissue

Most codes in Chapter 13 have site and laterality designations. The site designations for the limbs are the following:

- Upper arm
- Lower arm
- Upper and lower leg
    - Humerus
    - Ulna
    - Femur
    - Tibia
    - Fibula.

When a condition is described as *arm* or *leg* without further elaboration as to whether the site is upper or lower, the code for the upper arm or lower leg should be used. When the condition identifies more than one bone, joint, or muscle, a code for multiple sites is selected. If a multiple site code is not available, and multiple sites are involved, each site is coded separately.

For example, a patient was treated by an orthopedic surgeon for osteoarthritis of the right knee. The patient complained of chronic knee pain that worsened at night. The physician prescribed an anti-inflammatory drug to relieve the pain. Using ICD-10-CM, the encounter is coded as M17.11 (Unilateral primary osteoarthritis, right knee).

DOCUMENTATION TIP

When both decubitus and nondecubitus ulcers are being coded, the site and depth must be documented in the medical record.

In another example, a patient was diagnosed with a ganglion of the left ankle and foot. The correct code is a six-character combination code, M67.472 (Ganglion, left ankle and foot).

In a final example, a 70-year-old patient was diagnosed with rheumatoid myopathy with rheumatoid arthritis of the right and left hips. In ICD-10-CM, there is no combination code in this category or code for multiple sites, so both codes are reported for the right and left hips:

M05.451   Rheumatoid myopathy with rheumatoid arthritis of right hip

M05.452   Rheumatoid myopathy with rheumatoid arthritis of left hip

Many conditions in Chapter 13 of ICD-10-CM are results of trauma or previous injury to a site or are recurrent conditions. A current acute injury is reported with an injury code. Also included in this chapter are recurrent bone, joint, and muscle conditions.

Osteoporosis is also coded in Chapter 13 in ICD-10-CM. The two categories of codes are as follows:

M80   Osteoporosis with current pathological fracture

M81   Osteoporosis without current pathological fracture

Osteoporosis is a systemic condition in which all bones of the musculoskeletal system are affected. Category M81 is reported for patients who do not currently have a pathological fracture resulting from the osteoporosis but may have had a pathological fracture in the past. For patients with a history of fractures as a result of osteoporosis, status code Z87.31 (Personal history of [healed] osteoporosis fracture) is reported. Category M80 is reported for a patient who has a current pathological fracture. A traumatic fracture code is not reported for a patient with known osteoporosis who suffers a fracture, even if the patient has a minor fall or trauma, if that fall would not usually break a normal, healthy bone. Review Figure 7.25, which is an example from ICD-10-CM for osteoporosis without pathological fracture.

FIGURE 7.25 Excerpt From ICD-10-CM Tabular List, M81 and Z87.31

M81   Osteoporosis without current pathological fracture
  Use additional code to identify:
   major osseous defect, if applicable (M89.7-)
   personal history of osteoporosis fracture (Z87.31)
  Excludes1: osteoporosis with current pathological fracture (M80.-),
    Sudeck's atrophy (M89.0)

 M81.0   Age-related osteoporosis without current pathological fracture
   Involutional osteoporosis without current pathological fracture
   Osteoporosis NOS
   Postmenopausal osteoporosis without current pathological
    fracture
   Senile osteoporosis without current pathological fracture

FIGURE 7.25 **Excerpt From ICD-10-CM Tabular List, M81 and Z87.31** *(continued)*

M81.6   Localized osteoporosis [Lequesne]
  Excludes1: Sudeck's atrophy (M89.0)

M81.8   Other osteoporosis without current pathological fracture

  Drug-induced osteoporosis without current pathological fracture

  Idiopathic osteoporosis without current pathological fracture

  Osteoporosis of disuse without current pathological fracture

  Postoophorectomy osteoporosis without current pathological
   fracture

  Postsurgical malabsorption osteoporosis without current
   pathological fracture

  Post-traumatic osteoporosis without current pathological fracture

Z87.31   Personal history of (healed) osteoporosis fracture

DOCUMENTATION TIP

Code the personal history of a healed osteoporosis fracture using Z98.31.

For example, a patient was treated with medication for postmenopausal osteoporosis. The patient had a pathological fracture one year earlier, and the physician was seeing her in follow-up every three months. The ICD-10-CM coding is as follows:

Principal/first listed diagnosis–M81.0   Age-related osteoporosis without current pathological fracture

Secondary diagnosis–Z87.310   Personal history of (healed) osteoporosis fracture

Chapter 14 – Diseases of the Genitourinary System

Chronic kidney failure has three categories in ICD-10-CM:

N17   Acute kidney failure

N18   Chronic kidney disease

N19   Unspecified kidney failure

Chronic kidney disease is classified based on severity. Severity is designated using stages I to V. End-stage renal disease is coded when the provider has supported it in the medical record.

Category N19 is a nonspecific code that should be used rarely in the inpatient setting. Uremia NOS is classified in category N19. More precise information should be documented in the medical record to avoid using category N19.

Category N17 may be used as the principal diagnosis or as a secondary diagnosis. The diagnosis of acute kidney failure indicates the underlying condition that requires immediate attention. Sequencing is based on the underlying condition and focus of treatment. A code from N17 should always accompany a code for the causal condition. An instructional note following N17 specifies coding for the underlying condition.

Some common conditions of acute renal failure are dehydration and urinary obstruction. The acute renal failure should be reported first in these two conditions, if the focus of treatment is dehydration or urinary obstruction. Otherwise, the underlying condition should be sequenced first. When the underlying condition is the focus of treatment, the underlying condition is reported first, and the acute renal failure is sequenced as a secondary code. A code in category N17 should always include a code for the causal condition.

For example, a patient was admitted to the hospital with renal tubular necrosis. The patient was dehydrated and required intravenous fluid therapy for rehydration. Coding is as follows:

Principal/first listed diagnosis–N17.0	Acute renal failure with tubular necrosis
Secondary diagnosis–E86.0	Dehydration

In another example, a patient was admitted to the hospital with severe sepsis complicated by medullary necrosis. The coding is as follows:

Principal/first listed diagnosis–R65.20	Severe sepsis without septic shock
Secondary diagnosis–N17.2	Acute renal failure with medullary necrosis

In the example above, because the treatment is directed at the severe sepsis, the sepsis is listed first, followed by the acute renal failure.

Chronic kidney disease is malfunctioning of the kidneys resulting from such conditions as diabetes mellitus and hypertension or from drugs or chemicals that damage the kidneys. Chronic kidney disease is nonreversible. Treatment includes hemodialysis or peritoneal dialysis. Chronic kidney disease is not usually the reason for inpatient admission unless the patient is admitted for kidney transplantation. When a patient is receiving dialysis or any associated care, a code from category Z49 is reported as the first listed diagnosis, followed by a code from category N18. If a combination code exists to identify the chronic renal failure, a code from category N18 is not reported. If both a stage of chronic kidney disease and end-stage renal disease are documented, code N18.6 (End-stage renal disease) is the only code assigned. Kidney transplant status is reported with Z94.0, along with a code for the chronic kidney disease. Code N18- is used when the patient still has some form of chronic kidney disease. A transplant does not always restore kidney function.

For example, a patient with end-stage renal disease was admitted for dialysis. The patient was prepared and fitted for a peritoneal dialysis catheter, and dialysis was performed in the outpatient hospital dialysis center. The codes are as follows:

Principal/first listed diagnosis–Z49.02   Encounter for fitting and adjustment of peritoneal dialysis catheter

Secondary diagnosis–N18.6   End-stage renal disease

Chronic kidney disease requiring chronic dialysis.

A note after N18.6 instructs the user to report Z99.2 for dialysis status.

Tertiary diagnosis–Z99.2   Dependence on renal dialysis; hemodialysis status

Category N40 is reported for hyperplasia of the prostate gland, which includes combination codes for both the prostate gland condition and any associated complications. It is not necessary, unless directed, to use additional codes associated with the code for hyperplasia of the prostate gland.

For example, a patient saw a urologist with a complaint of urinary urgency and was diagnosed with hyperplasia of the prostate gland with urinary obstruction. Review Figure 7.26.

FIGURE 7.26 Excerpt From ICD-10-CM Tabular List, N40

N40   Enlarged prostate (EP)

        Includes: Adenofibromatous hypertrophy of prostate

                Benign hypertrophy of the prostate

                Benign prostatic hyperplasia

                Benign prostatic hypertrophy (BPH)

                Nodular prostate

                Polyp of prostate

        Excludes2: benign neoplasms of prostate (adenoma, benign) (fibroadenoma), (fibroma) (myoma) (D29.1) malignant neoplasm of prostate (C61)

    N40.0   Enlarged prostate without lower urinary tract symptoms(LUTS)

              Enlarged prostate NOS

    N40.1   Enlarged prostate with lower urinary tract symptoms (LUTS)

              Use additional code for associated symptoms, when specified:

                incomplete bladder emptying (R39.14)

                nocturia (R35.1)

                straining on urination (R39.16)

                urinary frequency (R35.0)

                urinary hesitancy (R39.11)

                urinary incontinence (N39.4-)

                urinary obstruction (N13.8)

                urinary retention (R33.8)

                urinary urgency (R39.15)

                weak urinary stream (R39.12)

The principal/first listed diagnosis is N40.1, Enlarged prostate with lower urinary tract symptoms (LUTS). The secondary diagnosis is R39.15, Urgency of urination. Review the comparison between ICD-9-CM and ICD-10-CM in Figure 7.27.

DOCUMENTATION TIP

Report Z99.2 for dialysis status.

FIGURE 7.27 **Comparison Between ICD-9-CM and ICD-10-CM for Coding of Enlarged Prostate Gland**

ICD-9-CM		ICD-10-CM	
600.91	Hyperplasia of prostate, unspecified, with urinary obstruction and other lower urinary tract symptoms (LUTS)	N40.1	Enlarged prostate with lower urinary tract symptoms (LUTS)
788.63	Urinary urgency	R39.15	Urgency of urination

Chapter 15 – Pregnancy, Childbirth, and the Puerperium

Chapter 15 includes codes for obstetric patients. The first obstetric code assigned should be based on the reason for the patient encounter. The first assigned diagnosis should be the reason for the encounter. Codes in this classification range from O00-O99. Chapter 15 codes have sequencing priority over codes from other chapters. Additional codes from other chapters may be reported to further report the patient's condition.

Pregnancy incidental is reported as Z33.1 (pregnancy state, incidental) and is used when the condition treated is not affecting the pregnancy. For example, if a patient is treated by the obstetrician for acute maxillary sinusitis, it is most likely that the condition will not affect the pregnancy. The patient encounter is reported as follows:

Primary/first listed diagnosis–J01.0   Acute maxillary sinusitis
Secondary diagnosis–Z33.1   Pregnancy state, incidental

For patient encounters in which no delivery occurs, the most significant complication of pregnancy should be sequenced first, if more than one complication occurs. When delivery occurs, the principal/first listed diagnosis should correspond to the main complication or circumstance of delivery. When cesarean delivery occurs, the principal/first listed diagnosis should correspond to the reason the cesarean delivery was performed unless the reason is unrelated to the condition resulting in the cesarean delivery.

The majority of the codes beginning with category O09 identify a final character indicating the trimester of pregnancy. Time frames of trimester are provided at the beginning of the chapter. This differs from ICD-9-CM. Trimesters are counted from the first day of the last menstrual period. Trimesters are defined as follows:

First trimester: less than 14 weeks 0 days

Second trimester: 14 weeks 0 days to less than 28 weeks 0 days

Third trimester: 28 weeks 0 days until delivery

Codes for unspecified trimester should never be reported unless it is impossible to determine the trimester from the documentation in the medical record. Routine normal pregnancy is reported as Z34- (Encounter for supervision of normal pregnancy). The fourth character identifies whether the pregnancy is the first pregnancy, using a fourth character (0); other normal pregnancy (8), or unspecified normal pregnancy (9). The fifth character identifies the trimester.

For example, a patient in the third trimester of her first pregnancy was seen for a routine visit. The patient was doing well, maintaining a healthy diet, and getting daily exercise. The encounter would be coded as follows: Primary/first listed diagnosis–Z34.03, Encounter for supervision of normal first pregnancy, third trimester.

For a patient who is receiving prenatal care for a high-risk pregnancy, a code from O09- is reported for supervision of a high-risk pregnancy. A secondary diagnosis code may be reported to identify any additional conditions present. Review Figure 7.28.

FIGURE 7.28 Excerpt From ICD-10-CM Tabular List, O09.7

O09.7   Supervision of high-risk pregnancy due to social problems

    O09.70   Supervision of high-risk pregnancy due to social problems, unspecified trimester

    O09.71   Supervision of high-risk pregnancy due to social problems, first trimester

    O09.72   Supervision of high-risk pregnancy due to social problems, second trimester

    O09.73   Supervision of high-risk pregnancy due to social problems, third trimester

---

If a trimester character is not provided for a specific code in the category, it is because the condition always occurs in a specific trimester or the trimester is not applicable, such as postpartum care. Review the following example and Figure 7.29: A patient with gestational diabetes was seen by the obstetrician for a routine visit during her seventh month of pregnancy. The patient was doing well and her gestational diabetes was well controlled with diet.

FIGURE 7.29 Excerpt From ICD-10-CM Tabular List, O24.4

O24.4   Gestational diabetes mellitus
      Diabetes mellitus arising in pregnancy
      Gestational diabetes mellitus NOS
     O24.41   Gestational diabetes mellitus in pregnancy
         O24.410   Gestational diabetes mellitus in pregnancy, diet controlled
         O24.414   Gestational diabetes mellitus in pregnancy, insulin controlled
         O24.419   Gestational diabetes mellitus in pregnancy, unspecified control
     O24.42   Gestational diabetes mellitus in childbirth
         O24.420   Gestational diabetes mellitus in childbirth, diet controlled
         O24.424   Gestational diabetes mellitus in childbirth, insulin controlled
         O24.429   Gestational diabetes mellitus in childbirth, unspecified control
     O24.43   Gestational diabetes mellitus in the puerperium
         O24.430   Gestational diabetes mellitus in the puerperium, diet controlled
         O24.434   Gestational diabetes mellitus in the puerperium, insulin controlled
         O24.439   Gestational diabetes mellitus in the puerperium, unspecified control

---

The correct code is reported as O24.410 for the gestional diabetes mellitus in pregnancy, diet controlled. When a patient is admitted to the hospital because of complications of pregnancy and remains in the hospital for antepartum, delivery, and postpartum complications, the final character that corresponds to the trimester of the occurrence of the complication should be used. It is also acceptable to use codes indicating different trimesters of pregnancy as well as postpartum care on the same record. When a patient has gestational diabetes and is treated with both diet and insulin, the default is for insulin controlled. When a patient has diabetes mellitus and becomes pregnant, a code from O24- is assigned along with a code for diabetes (E08–E13).

Complications of etopic pregnancy, miscarriage, and other abnormal products of conception are coded in Chapter 15. Complications category blocks include the following:

O00   Etopic pregnancy

O01   Hydatidiform mole

O02   Other abnormal products of conception

O03   Spontaneous abortion

All codes in these blocks require a code from category O08 (Complications following ectopic and molar pregnancy) to identify the complication. If the encounter is for the complication after the initial patient encounter or the pregnancy, only a code from O08 should be reported.

For example, a patient was treated for defibrination syndrome following an ectopic pregnancy that occurred three weeks earlier. The following codes should be reported:

O08.1   Delayed or excessive hemorrhage following ectopic and molar pregnancy

            Defibrination syndrome following ectopic and molar pregnancy

Coding for Multiple Gestations

Multiple gestations are coded using blocks beginning with O30-. An extension is added to codes for multiple gestations indicating which fetus is affected by a particular condition or code. This is different from coding in ICD-9-CM, which does not have a code for identifying the complication based on which fetus is affected. See Figure 7.30.

FIGURE 7.30 **Excerpt From ICD-10-CM Tabular List, O30.1**

O30.1	Triplet pregnancy	
	O30.10	Triplet pregnancy, unspecified trimester
	O30.11	Triplet pregnancy, first trimester
	O30.12	Triplet pregnancy, second trimester
	O30.13	Triplet pregnancy, third trimester

One of the following seventh characters is to be assigned to each code under category O31:

0:   Single gestations and multiple gestations in which the fetus is unspecified

1-9:   Cases of multiple gestations in which the identity of the fetus for which the code applies is specified

The appropriate code from category O30, Multiple gestation, must also be assigned when a code that has a seventh character of one through nine is assigned from category O31. Review the character extensions.

0:   not applicable or unspecified
1:   fetus 1
2:   fetus 2
3:   fetus 3
4:   fetus 4
5:   fetus 5
9:   other fetus

Review Figure 7.31 for an example of category O31.3 for a patient continuing pregnancy after spontaneous abortion of one or more fetuses.

FIGURE 7.31 Excerpt From ICD-10-CM Tabular List, O31.3

O31.3   Continuing pregnancy after elective fetal reduction of one fetus or more
       Continuing pregnancy after selective termination of one fetus or more
     O31.30   Continuing pregnancy after elective fetal reduction of one fetus or more, unspecified trimester
     O31.31   Continuing pregnancy after elective fetal reduction of one fetus or more, first trimester
     O31.32   Continuing pregnancy after elective fetal reduction of one fetus or more, second trimester
     O31.33   Continuing pregnancy after elective fetal reduction of one fetus or more, third trimester

---

For example, a patient in the second trimester of pregnancy with six fetuses underwent surgery to reduce the fetuses to five in hopes of survival of the other fetuses. The first listed diagnosis is O31.321 (Continuing pregnancy after elective fetal reduction of one fetus or more, second trimester). Note that the seventh character extension is *1*, because only one fetus is reduced.

An ectopic pregnancy coded in category O00 that occurs with an intrauterine pregnancy is considered a multiple gestation. Both the ectopic pregnancy and intrauterine pregnancy should be reported with an extension. Any complication resulting from the ectopic pregnancy (O08) should be reported with the same extension as O00. All codes for intrauterine pregnancy should have the same extension to distinguish them from the ectopic pregnancy codes.

HIV in a Pregnant Patient

HIV in a pregnant patient is reported with O98.7- when a patient has an HIV infection or HIV-related illness. That code is followed by the appropriate HIV code for the disease. Review Figure 7.32.

FIGURE 7.32 Excerpt From ICD-10-CM Tabular List, O98.7

O98.7   Human immunodeficiency [HIV] disease complicating pregnancy, childbirth, and the puerperium
     Use additional code to identify the type of HIV disease:
        Acquired immune deficiency syndrome (AIDS) (B20)
        Asymptomatic HIV status (Z21)
        HIV positive NOS (Z21)
        Symptomatic HIV disease (B20)
     O98.71   Human immunodeficiency [HIV] disease complicating pregnancy

> **FIGURE 7.32 Excerpt From ICD-10-CM Tabular List, O98.7** *(continued)*
>
> O98.711 Human immunodeficiency [HIV] disease complicating pregnancy, first trimester
>
> O98.712 Human immunodeficiency [HIV] disease complicating pregnancy, second trimester
>
> O98.713 Human immunodeficiency [HIV] disease complicating pregnancy, third trimester
>
> O98.719 Human immunodeficiency [HIV] disease complicating pregnancy, unspecified trimester
>
> O98.72 Human immunodeficiency [HIV] disease complicating childbirth
>
> O98.73 Human immunodeficiency [HIV] disease complicating the puerperium

For example, a patient in the second trimester of pregnancy was HIV positive. Her pregnancy was progressing well without complications. The coding is as follows:

Primary/first listed diangosis–O98.712   Human immunodeficiency [HIV] disease complicating pregnancy, second trimester

Secondary diagnosis–Z21   HIV positive NOS

Category O09 for supervision of high-risk pregnancy is coded in this category when the patient has had a complication with pregnancy during a current or a past pregnancy.

Normal Delivery

Normal delivery is reported with category O80- and is assigned for a patient who is admitted for a full-term normal delivery and delivers a single healthy infant without any antepartum complications, during delivery or postpartum during the delivery episode. Code O80- is always the first listed diagnosis. Other diagnoses may be reported if they are not related to or complicating the pregnancy.

Code O80- may also be used if the patient had a complication during the pregnancy, but the complication is not present at time of delivery. A high-risk pregnancy does not constitute a complication.

Outcome of delivery is reported with category Z37-. This category is intended to be used as an additional code to identify the outcome of delivery for the mother's record. It is not reported on the newborn record. Outcome of delivery is reported as a secondary code following the delivery code (O80-).

Review some examples of expanded codes for outcome of delivery in ICD-10-CM:

- Z37.0   Single live birth
- Z37.1   Single stillbirth
- Z37.2   Twins, both liveborn

- Z37.3   Twins, one liveborn and one stillborn
- Z37.4   Twins, both stillborn
- Z37.5   Other multiple births, all liveborn
- Z37.50   Multiple births, unspecified, all liveborn
- Z37.51   Triplets, all liveborn
- Z37.52   Quadruplets, all liveborn
- Z37.53   Quintuplets, all liveborn
- Z73.54   Sextuplets, all liveborn
- Z37.59   Other multiple births, all liveborn

> **DOCUMENTATION TIP**
>
> Codes Z37- (Outcome of delivery) are reported only on the mother's record, not on the infant's record.

Chapter 16 – Certain Conditions Originating in the Newborn (Perinatal Period)

The perinatal period covers birth through the 28th day. Any clinically significant condition noted on the newborn examination is coded, with the most serious and requiring the most care reported first. A condition is considered clinically significant if it involves the following:

- Clinical evaluation
- Therapeutic treatment
- Diagnostic procedure
- Extended length of hospital stay
- Increased nursing care or monitoring
- Implications for future health care needs.

Codes in Chapter 16 are used only for the newborn or infant and not on the maternal record. Codes in this chapter are also applicable only to liveborn infants. If the condition continues through the life of the child, regardless of the age of the patient, it should be coded. If the condition may be due to the birth process or be community acquired, the default should be the *Complication at birth* code(s) from Chapter 16. These conditions are codes from blocks P35 to P39, based on the infection or condition.

For example, a newborn was diagnosed with congenital viral hepatitis by the pediatrician. The encounter is coded as P35.3 (Congenital viral hepatitis). Review Figure 7.33.

FIGURE 7.33 Excerpt From ICD-10-CM Tabular List, P35

P35   Congenital viral diseases
     Includes: infections acquired in utero or during birth
    P35.0   Congenital rubella syndrome
         Congenital rubella pneumonitis
    P35.1   Congenital cytomegalovirus infection
    P35.2   Congenital herpes viral [herpes simplex] infection
    P35.3   Congenital viral hepatitis
    P35.8   Other congenital viral diseases
         Congenital varicella [chickenpox]
    P35.9   Congenital viral disease, unspecified

When a newborn is suspected to have a problem because of the condition of the mother, categories P00 to P04 are reported. Codes for *Newborns affected by maternal factors and complications of pregnancy, labor, and delivery* are used for these encounters. If tests or treatment are performed, codes in this category are used. In addition, if the problem is confirmed, a code for the condition is reported, followed by a code from P00 to P04.

For example, a two-day-old baby was suspected to be in drug withdrawal. The neonate's mother was an active cocaine user up until delivery. The encounter is coded as P04.41, Newborn (suspected to be) affected by maternal use of cocaine.

Prematurity, Low Birth Weight, and Immaturity Status

- P05.-   Disorders of newborn related to slow fetal growth and fetal malnutrition
- P07.-   Disorders of newborn related to short gestation and low birth weight, not elsewhere classified
- P07.10 Other low birth weight newborn, specify birth weight
- P07.2   Extreme immaturity of newborn
- P07.3   Other preterm newborn, specify weight of gestation
- Z38.-   Liveborn infants according to place of birth and type of delivery

Review some examples of reporting birth weight for small newborns in ICD-10-CM.

- P05.10 Newborn small for gestational age, unspecified weight
- P05.11 Newborn small for gestational age, less than 500 grams
- P05.12 Newborn small for gestational age, 500-749 grams
- P05.13 Newborn small for gestational age, 750-999 grams
- P05.14 Newborn small for gestational age, 1000-1249 grams
- P05.15 Newborn small for gestational age, 1250-1499 grams
- P05.16 Newborn small for gestational age, 1500-1749 grams
- P05.17 Newborn small for gestational age, 1750-1999 grams
- P05.18 Newborn small for gestational age, 2000-2499 grams

GUIDELINE TIP

Code Z91.71 is reported for a child or an adult who was small as a newborn.

Liveborn Status

Codes for liveborn infants according to place of birth is coded with category Z38. This code is used as the principal diagnosis on the initial birth record and is not reported on the mother's record. Review some examples for reporting live born infants according to place of birth and method of delivery.

- Z38.0   Single liveborn infant, born in hospital
- Z38.00 Single liveborn infant, delivered vaginally
- Z38.01 Single liveborn infant, delivered by cesarean
- Z38.1   Single liveborn infant, born outside hospital
- Z38.2   Single liveborn infant, unspecified as to place of birth
- Z38.3   Twin liveborn infant, born in hospital
- Z38.30 Twin liveborn infant, delivered vaginally

- Z38.31   Twin liveborn infant, delivered by cesarean
- Z38.4   Twin liveborn infant, born outside hospital
- Z38.5   Twin liveborn infant, unspecified as to place of birth

Chapter 17 – Congenital Malformations, Deformations, and Chromosomal Abnormalities

Codes in this category may be used for any patient, regardless of age. Blocks in this category include the following:

- Q00–Q07   Congenital malformations of the nervous system
- Q10–Q18   Congenital malformations of the eye, ear, face, and neck
- Q20–Q28   Congenital malformations of the circulatory system
- Q30–Q34   Congenital malformations of the respiratory system
- Q35–Q37   Cleft lip and cleft palate
- Q38–Q45   Other congenital malformations of the digestive system
- Q50–Q56   Congenital malformations of the genital organs
- Q60–Q64   Congenital malformations of the urinary system
- Q65–Q79   Congenital malformations and deformations of the muscu-
            loskeletal system
- Q80–Q89   Other congenital malformations
- Q90–Q99   Chromosomal abnormalities, not elsewhere classified.

Three new categories not found in ICD-9-CM were added to Chapter 17 of ICD-10-CM:

- Q11.3   Macrophthalmos
- Q20.6   Isomerism of atrial appendages
- Q22.6   Hypoplastic right heart syndrome.

Congenital anomalies or syndromes may occur as a set of symptoms or multiple malformations. If there is no code for a syndrome, for every manifestation of that syndrome, a code should be reported from any chapter in the classification. If there is a specific code to identify the congenital anomaly or syndrome, additional codes may be assigned to identify manifestations not included in the code for the syndrome.

Chapter 18 – Symptoms, Signs, and Abnormal Clinical and Laboratory Findings, Not Elsewhere Classified

This chapter includes codes for symptoms, signs, abnormal results of clinical or other investigative procedures, and ill-defined conditions. Codes are assigned when no diagnosis has been made that can be classified elsewhere. If a definitive diagnosis cannot be determined, a sign/symptom code is reported, as in ICD-9-CM. If a confirmed diagnosis is documented in the medical record, only the confirmed diagnosis is reported unless the sign/symptom is not related to the definitive diagnosis.

Many codes in this chapter are combination codes that include the diagnosis and the most common symptoms of that diagnosis. When a combination code is the appropriate code to report, a secondary code is not reported for the symptom.

For example, a patient visited his family physician with symptoms of nausea and vomiting. The symptoms began two days earlier. The patient had no other symptoms. The physician examined the patient and prescribed medication to help with the condition. Review the coding comparison between ICD-9-CM and ICD-10-CM for this situation in Figure 7.34.

FIGURE 7.34 **Comparison Between ICD-9-CM and ICD-10-CM for Coding of Symptoms**

ICD-9-CM		ICD-10-CM	
787.0	Nausea and vomiting	R11	Nausea and vomiting
787.01	Nausea with vomiting		Excludes1:
			cyclical vomiting associated with migraine (G43.81-)
787.02	Nausea alone		excessive vomiting in pregnancy (O21.-)
787.03	Vomiting alone		hematemesis (K92.0)
			neonatal hematemesis (P54.0)
			newborn vomiting (P92.0)
			psychogenic vomiting (F50.8)
			vomiting following gastrointestinal surgery (K91.0)
		R11.0	Nausea without vomiting
		R11.1	Vomiting
		R11.10	Vomiting unspecified
		R11.11	Vomiting without nausea
		R11.12	Projectile vomiting
		R11.13	Vomiting of fecal matter
		R11.14	Bilious vomiting
		R11.2	Nausea with vomiting, unspecified

Notice in Figure 7.34 that ICD-9-CM does not have a code for projectile vomiting or other vomiting without nausea. There are specific codes in ICD-10-CM that includes projectile vomiting (R11.2) as well as other vomiting without nausea (R11.3).

Some of the block and category titles have been changed in Chapter 18, as have titles in other chapters in ICD-10-CM. For example, category 786 (Symptoms involving respiratory systems and other chest symptoms) in ICD-9-CM is changed in ICD-10-CM to R06 (Abnormalities of breathing).

For example, a patient with chest pain and shortness of breath on exertion was seen by a cardiologist. The physician documented a diagnosis of bradycardia. Review the comparison between ICD-9-CM and ICD-10-CM coding in Figure 7.35.

FIGURE 7.35 Comparison Between ICD-9-CM and ICD-10-CM for Coding of Bradycardia

ICD-9-CM		ICD-10-CM	
427.89	Other specified cardiac dysrhythmias	R00.1	Bradycardia, unspecified

Other examples of new ICD-10-CM category codes include the following:
- R33   Retention of urine
- R58   Hemorrhage, not elsewhere classified
- R77   Other abnormalities of plasma proteins
- R78   Finding of drugs and other substances, not normally found in blood

The codes for abnormal findings have been significantly expanded in ICD-10-CM to provide greater specificity. The block entitled *Abnormal findings on examination of other body fluids, substances and tissues, without diagnosis* includes the following categories:
- R83   Abnormal findings in cerebrospinal fluid
- R84   Abnormal findings in specimens from respiratory organs and thorax
- R85   Abnormal findings in specimens from digestive organs and abdominal cavity
- R86   Abnormal findings in specimens from male genital organs
- R87   Abnormal findings in specimens from female genital organs
- R88   Abnormal findings in other body fluids and substances
- R89   Abnormal findings in specimens from other organs, systems, and tissues.

Falling

Other abnormalities of gait and mobility are to be used when the patient tends to fall when attempting to walk and should not be confused with the external-cause codes for falls.
- R26.8   Other abnormalities of gait and mobility
- R26.81   Unsteadiness on feet.

This code category may be used in conjunction with the external-cause codes for falls. The injury codes are reported first, followed by the underlying condition and the external-cause code to describe the type of fall. Repeated falls are reported as R29.6 when the patient has recently fallen and the reason for the fall is under investigation.

Glasgow Coma Scale

According to the coding guidelines for ICD-10-CM, the Glasgow coma scale must be used in conjunction with the codes for traumatic brain injuries or the sequelae of cerebrovascular accidents. With code R40.2-, one code from each of the three subcategories must be assigned to complete the Glasgow coma scale. When more than one coma assessment is performed (multiple coma assessments), the patient's health record should include a report of the initial coma scale performed at the time of admission and a final rating performed at the time of discharge.

Facility policy should determine which scale ratings are to be reported in the health record. A seven character extension must be added to the coma codes to indicate which ratings are to be reported in the final record.

In ICD-9-CM, the correct code for coma is 780.01, with no additional specificity. ICD-10-CM has expanded the codes for coma. Review this expanded code category. It is evident that more information must be documented in the medical record to code in this category in ICD-10-CM (see Figure 7.36).

DOCUMENTATION TIP

In ICD-10-CM, coma is coded on the basis of a coma scale.

FIGURE 7.36 Excerpt From ICD-10-CM Tabular List, R40.2-

R40.2   Coma

Coma NOS

Unconsciousness NOS

Code first any associated:

coma in fracture of skull (S02.–)

coma in intracranial injury (S06.–)

The following seventh character extensions are to be added to codes R40.21, R40.22, R40.23

0   unspecified time

1   in the field [EMT or ambulance]

2   at arrival to emergency department

3   at hospital admission

4   24 hours after hospital admission

A code from each subcategory is required to complete the coma scale.

R40.20   Unspecified coma

R40.21   Coma scale, eyes open

R40.211   Coma scale, eyes open, never

R40.212   Coma scale, eyes open, to pain

R40.213   Coma scale, eyes open, to sound

R40.214   Coma scale, eyes open, spontaneous

Note: These codes are intended primarily for trauma registry and research but may be utilized by all users of the classification who wish to collect this information.

FIGURE 7.36 Excerpt From ICD-10-CM Tabular List, R40.2- *(continued)*

R40.22   Coma scale, best verbal response
      R40.221   Coma scale, best verbal response, none
      R40.222   Coma scale, best verbal response, incomprehensible words
      R40.223   Coma scale, best verbal response, inappropriate words
      R40.224   Coma scale, best verbal response, confused conversation
      R40.225   Coma scale, best verbal response, oriented

R40.23   Coma scale, best motor response
      R40.231   Coma scale, best motor response, none
      R40.232   Coma scale, best motor response, extension
      R40.233   Coma scale, best motor response, abnormal
      R40.234   Coma scale, best motor response, flexion withdrawal
      R40.235   Coma scale, best motor response, localizes pain
      R40.236   Coma scale, best motor response, obeys commands

---

Summary

This chapter includes coding guidelines and clarification for coding in various chapters using ICD-10-CM. It is important to review changes to the *ICD-10-CM Official Guidelines for Coding and Reporting, 2009* on a yearly basis prior to and after implementation as well as to review the chapters that will impact implementation plans as the practice moves forward to ICD-10-CM migration.

Resources

ICD-10-CM Official Guidelines for Coding and Reporting, 2009. Available online at ftp://ftp.cdc.gov/pub/Health_Statistics/NCHS/Publications/ICD10CM/2009/.

National Center for Health Statistics. *ICD-10-CM Tabular List.* Available online at ftp://ftp.cdc.gov/pub/Health_Statistics/NCHS/Publications/ICD10CM/2009/.

End-of-Chapter Questions

1 In ICD-9-CM, diseases of the eye and adnexa are located with

_____ system, but in ICD-10-CM, the codes

are located in Chapter _____.

2 Codes for hypertensive heart disease in ICD-10-CM are found in

what categories? _____

3 How is secondary hypertension reported in ICD-10-CM? _____

_____

_____

4 If a patient has multiple complications of Crohn's disease _____

_____ may be reported from _____ or _____ for each
complication.

5 When coma is being coded in ICD-10-CM, what must be used in
conjunction with the coma codes for brain injuries or the sequelae of
cerebrovascular accidents? _____

CHAPTER 8

ICD-10-CM: Chapter-Specific Guidelines for Chapters 19 to 21

OBJECTIVES

* Understand chapter-specific guidelines for ICD-10-CM Chapters 19 to 21
* Review examples of ICD-10-CM codes relative to the guidelines
* Review comparisons between ICD-9-CM and ICD-10-CM

Introduction

This chapter covers chapter-specific guidelines in ICD-10-CM for the following:
* Chapter 19 – Injury, poisoning, and certain other consequences of external causes
* Chapter 20 – External causes of morbidity
* Chapter 21 – Factors influencing health status and contact with health services.

Chapter-Specific Guidelines

Chapter 19 – Injury, Poisoning, and Certain Other Consequences of External Causes

Chapter 19 includes S codes and T codes. S codes are used to report traumatic injuries. T codes report burns and corrosions, poisonings and toxic effects, adverse effects, underdosing, complications of medical care, and other such consequences of external causes.

Most blocks in this chapter require a seventh character extension for the applicable code. Most categories use three extensions.

A Initial encounter
D Subsequent encounter
S Sequela

Fractures are reported with different extensions. Extension *a* is used only for the first patient encounter for the treatment of an injury. All subsequent encounters require extension *d*. An injury code with extension *d* may be used as long as the patient is treated for the injury for the entire course of treatment for a specific injury. Even if the patient delays seeking treatment, the first encounter with the provider is considered the initial encounter. However, if another medical professional has treated the patient previously for the injury, the encounter is coded as subsequent treatment. If the nature of the encounter is unknown, it is reported with extension *a* for initial treatment.

Extension *s* is used for complications or conditions as a direct result of an injury. A good example is scar formation following a burn. The scars would be sequelae of the burn. The ICD-10-CM guidelines direct the user to report the injury code that precipitated the complication and the code for the sequela.

The *s* is added to the injury code, not the code for the complication or sequela. The sequela is sequenced first (complication or the condition as a result of the injury) and the injury code is sequenced secondarily.

Injury codes or S codes are reported for injuries. The most severe injury is sequenced first. Injury codes are categorized by type of injury and site. There are instructional notes to indicate which other codes are used to fully describe the injury. For open wounds, for example, an instructional note provides guidance to the user to code any associated wound infection. For normal healing surgical wounds, a wound code in this chapter is not used.

Codes in this category are divided into body regions:

- S00-S09   Injuries to the head
- S10-S19   Injuries to the neck
- S20-S29   Injuries to the thorax
- S30-S39   Injuries to the abdomen, lower back, lumbar spine, and pelvis
- S40-S49   Injuries to the shoulder and upper arm
- S50-S59   Injuries to the elbow and forearm
- S60-S69   Injuries to the wrist and hand
- S70-S79   Injuries to the hip
- S80-S89   Injuries to the knee and lower leg
- S90-S99   Injuries to the ankle and foot.

Within body section divisions are categories for type of injury specific to the body section. When coding superficial and open wounds, assign codes based on terms documented in the medical record. For example, if a wound is classified as a bite, it would be classified as an open bite. As with ICD-9-CM, superficial wounds are not coded with a more severe injury if it is associated with that injury at the same site.

For example, a patient who was not wearing a seat belt was involved in an automobile accident. He hit the windshield and was treated in the emergency department for a laceration to the scalp. Review the comparison to ICD-9-CM in Figure 8.1.

FIGURE 8.1 Comparison Between ICD-9-CM and ICD-10-CM for Coding of Scalp Laceration

ICD-9-CM		ICD-10-CM	
873.0	Other open wound of head, scalp without mention of complication	S01.01xA	Laceration without foreign body of scalp

---

The seventh character extension *A* would be reported because treatment is the reason for the initial encounter. As with ICD-9-CM, superficial injuries such as abrasions or contusions are not coded when associated with a more severe injury. If a primary injury results in major damage to peripheral nerves or blood vessels, the primary injury is sequenced as the first listed diagnosis, followed by an additional code for injury to the blood vessels. When the primary injury is to the blood vessels or nerves, that injury should be sequenced first.

Fracture Coding

Fractures are coded by site for each individual fracture. As many fracture codes as are needed to describe the fracture should be used, with the most serious fracture coded first. As with ICD-9-CM, a fracture not documented as open or closed is coded as closed. As with S codes, fracture codes include seventh character extensions *A, B, S,* in addition to additional extensions to identify whether the fracture is open or closed, for routine healing, delayed healing, nonunion, and malunion.

For open fractures of the long bones, extensions identify the degree of severity for the open fracture. The fracture extensions are unique to each type of bone and type of fracture. It is necessary to review the fracture extensions carefully before assigning an extension. A fracture code is reported for as long as the patient is receiving treatment for the fracture.

Review category S32 (Fracture of lumbar spine and pelvis), shown in Figure 8.2, and note the seventh character extensions added to this category.

FIGURE 8.2 Excerpt From ICD-10-CM Tabular List, S32

S32   Fracture of lumbar spine and pelvis

   A fracture not identified as displaced or nondisplaced should be coded
      to displaced

   Includes: fracture of lumbosacral neural arch
         fracture of lumbosacral spinous process
         fracture of lumbosacral transverse process
         fracture of lumbosacral vertebra
         fracture of lumbosacral vertebral arch

   Code first any associated spinal cord and spinal nerve injury (S34-)

   Excludes1: transection of abdomen (S38.3)

   Excludes2: fracture of hip NOS (S72.0-)

   The appropriate seventh character is to be added to each code from category S32

   A fracture not identified as open or closed should be coded to closed

   A   initial encounter for closed fracture
   B   initial encounter for open fracture
   D   subsequent encounter for fracture with routine healing
   G   subsequent encounter for fracture with delayed healing
   K   subsequent encounter for fracture with nonunion
   S   sequela

For example, a patient underwent surgery for an open burst fracture of the lumbar vertebra, which became unstable. The encounter is coded in ICD-10-CM as S32.012, Unstable burst fracture of first lumbar vertebra. A seventh character extension is required for this category. Because the documentation identifies this as an open fracture, the seventh character extension is *B*, initial encounter for open fracture. The encounter is then reported as S32.012B.

For aftercare of an injury, do not use a *Z* aftercare code; report the aftercare of an injury by assigning an acute injury code with the seventh digit extension *D* for subsequent encounter.

Crush injuries are sequenced first, followed by any code to indicate the specific injuries associated with the crushing. Review the following example: A patient was treated in an emergency department three days earlier for a crushing injury to the right hand that resulted from equipment falling on his hand at a construction site. The physician treated the patient and referred him to a hand surgeon. The hand surgeon evaluated the patient and determined that surgery was indicated.

The encounter is reported as S67.21B, Crushing injury of right hand. The seventh character extension *B* is applicable because another physician provided treatment for the initial encounter, and treatment by the hand surgeon is subsequent.

Amputations

If an amputation is not documented as partial or complete, it should be coded as a complete amputation. Amputation codes include the fracture of the bone, and the fracture code is not reported in addition to the code for the amputation.

Spinal Cord Injuries

For each section of spinal cord injury, the code for the highest level of injury for that section of the cord should be used. If a patient has a cord injury at more than one section of the cord, use a code for the highest level of injury for each section. If the patient has a complete lesion of the cord, it is not necessary to use any additional codes for spinal cord injuries below the level of the complete lesion.

External-cause codes are located in Chapter 20 of ICD-10-CM. When an injury code is reported, the cause of injury must also be assigned. The ICD-10-CM coding guidelines do not specify the external-cause codes as optional. The activity (Y93) and the place of occurrence (Y93-) should also be assigned. The guidelines state that place of occurrence is not required for adverse effects, poisonings, or toxic effects. Codes in this category must include a seventh character extension to identify what type of activity is performed. The seventh character extensions include the following:

1   non–work-related activity

2   work-related activity

3   student activity (activity performed not for income)

4   military activity.

If the injury is work related, a seventh character 2 should be added to the activity code. Place of occurrence codes are limited in ICD-9-CM but have been expanded in ICD-10-CM.

For example, while playing tennis in an amateur tournament at a country club, a female player sprained her right wrist and was treated in an urgent care center near the club. The principal/first listed diagnosis is S63.501A, Unspecified sprain of right wrist, initial encounter. The secondary diagnosis is Y93.025, Tennis (external cause, activity). The tertiary diagnosis is Y92.312, Tennis court as the place of occurrence of the external cause.

Burns and Corrosions

ICD-10-CM distinguishes between burns and corrosions. The burn codes are to report thermal burns that come from a heat source, such as a fire or hot appliance. The burn codes are also for burns resulting from electricity and radiation, whereas corrosions are burns due to chemicals.

If a burn is a thermal burn, a burn code should be used. If a burn is a chemical burn, a corrosion code should be used. The guidelines for burns and corrosions are the same. Sunburns are not coded in this category. Category T20 to T25 is used to report burns and corrosions.

These codes are classified by:

- site;
- depth; and
- degree: first degree, erythema; second degree, blistering; third degree, full thickness.

Burns of the eye (T26-T28) are classified by site, not degree. Each burn or corrosion site is coded by sequencing the highest degree of burn or corrosion when more than one site is affected. Internal burns and corrosions are reported before external burns, if they require more extensive treatment or are more severe. As with ICD-9-CM, code burns of the same site to the highest degree using one code, even if the burns or corrosions are of different degrees.

Coding Total Body Surface Area (TBSA) for Burns or Corrosions

For coding TBSA, an additional code is assigned to one of the following categories:

T31   Burns classified according to extent of body surface involved

T32   Corrosions classified according to extent of body surface involved

These codes are used to indicate the TBSA burned and should be reported when there is mention of a third degree burn involving 20% or more TBSA. These codes may be reported, if the TBSA is less than 20%.

Categories T31 and T32 are based on the classic *rule of nines* for estimating percentage of body surface involved: head and neck, 9%; each arm, 9%; each leg 9%; the anterior trunk, 18%; posterior trunk, 18%, and genitalia, 1%. Physicians may change these percentage assignments where necessary to accommodate infants and children who have proportionately larger heads than adults and patients who have large buttocks, thighs, or abdomens that involve burns or corrosions.

For example, a patient suffered a third degree burn of the trunk involving 10% TBSA, a second degree burn of the cheek, and a third degree burn of the forehead involving 4% TBSA during a house fire and was taken to an emergency department for treatment. Review the comparison between ICD-9-CM and ICD-10-CM for burn coding in Figure 8.3

FIGURE 8.3 Comparison Between ICD-9-CM and ICD-10-CM for Coding of Burns

ICD-9-CM		ICD-10-CM	
942.30	Burn of trunk, full thickness skin loss (third degree NOS), unspecified site	T21.30xA	Burn of third degree of trunk, unspecified site
941.37	Burn of face, head, and neck, full thickness skin loss (third degree NOS) forehead and cheek	T20.36xA	Burn of third degree of forehead and cheek
948.11	Burns classified according to extent of total body surface involved, 10-19%	T31.11xA	Burns involving 10-19% of body surface with 10-19% third degree burns

---

Nonhealing or infected burns and corrosions are reported as acute burns or corrosions. Necrosis of burned skin is coded as a nonhealed burn. An infection as the result of a burn (infected burn site) should be reported as an additional code. External-cause codes should be used with burns and corrosions to indicate the source of the burn, the place where it occurred, and the activity of the patient at the time of the incident.

Sequelae of Burns and Corrosions

Extension *s* should be assigned to a burn or corrosion code to indicate that a sequela of the burn or corrosion exists.

Poisonings, Toxic Effects, Adverse Effects, and Underdosing

ICD-10-CM does not provide codes that differentiate between poisonings and adverse effects. The various codes in the block T36 through T50 (Poisoning by, adverse effects of, and underdosing of drugs, medications, and biological substances) identify the substances that caused the adverse effect.

As with ICD-9-CM, a table of drugs and chemicals is available to assist in coding this category. When a nonprescribed drug or medicinal agent is taken in combination with a correctly prescribed and properly administered drug, any drug toxicity or other reaction resulting from the interaction of the two drugs is classified as a poisoning. When a drug prescribed is administered incorrectly, this is also considered a poisoning.

A toxic effect is a poisoning due to a toxic substance that has no medicinal use. An adverse effect is a reaction to a drug that is taken as prescribed and is properly administered.

Underdosing is taking less of a medication than is prescribed by a physician or the manufacturer's instruction with a resulting negative health consequence. A code for noncompliance (Z91.12-, Z91.13-) or a code for failure in dosage during surgical or medical care (Y63.-) must be used with an underdosing code to indicate intent. Review Figure 8.4 as an example of coding for underdosing.

FIGURE 8.4 Excerpt From ICD-10-CM Tabular List, Z91.12

Z91.12 Patient's intentional underdosing of medication regimen

   Code first underdosing of medication (T36-T50) with final character 6

   Excludes 1: adverse effect of prescribed drug taken as directed–code to adverse effect poisoning (overdose)–code to poisoning

      Z91.120   Patient's intentional underdosing of medication regimen due to financial hardship

---

Codes related to poisonings and certain other consequences of external causes are located in blocks T07 through T88. Category T07 (Unspecified multiple injuries) is to be used only when no documentation is available to identify the specific injuries. Code T07 would never be used in an inpatient setting.

As shown in Figure 8.5, categories T36 through T50 (Poisoning, adverse effects, and underdosing by drugs, medicaments and biological substances) and T51 through T65 (Toxic effects of substances chiefly nonmedicinal as to source) are the categories for the different classes of drugs and chemical agents that may cause a poisoning, toxic effect, or adverse effect.

FIGURE 8.5 Excerpt From ICD-10-CM Tabular List, T36

T36   Poisoning by, adverse effect of, and underdosing of systemic antibiotics

   T36.0   Poisoning by, adverse effect of, and underdosing of penicillins

      T36.0x1   Poisoning by penicillins, accidental (unintentional)

      T36.0x2   Poisoning by penicillins, intentional self-harm

      T36.0x3   Poisoning by penicillins, assault

      T36.0x4   Poisoning by penicillins, undetermined

      T36.0x5   Adverse effect of penicillins

      T36.0x6   Underdosing of penicillins

The user is directed to code to accidental poisoning when there is no intent indicated in the documentation. The code for undetermined intent should be used only when specific documentation in the record indicates that the intent could not be determined. Fifth and sixth characters indicate the circumstances that caused the adverse effect, such as accidental poisoning or adverse effect, intentional self-harm, assault, or undetermined cause.

Poisonings and toxic effects have an associated intent: accidental, intentional self-harm, assault, and undetermined. The final character code in these categories, usually the sixth character, indicates the intent. This is similar to coding poisonings and toxic effects in ICD-9-CM.

1 Accidental

2 Intentional (self-harm)

3 Assault

4 Undetermined

5 Adverse effects (categories T36-T50 only)

6 Underdosing (categories T36-T50 only)

No additional external-cause code is required for poisonings, toxic effects, adverse effects, and underdosing codes.

For example, a patient took an overdose of penicillin that was prescribed correctly, resulting in projectile vomiting. The primary/first listed diagnosis is T36.0x1A, Poisoning by penicillins, accidental (unintentional). The secondary diagnosis is R11.2, Projectile vomiting.

Poisonings, toxic effects, adverse effects, and underdosing are reported in different categories, as in ICD-9-CM. The ICD-9-CM Table of Drugs and Chemicals classifies poisonings and adverse effects separately. In ICD-10-CM, they are not separated into different categories but are coded within the same classification.

An example of the Table of Drugs and Chemicals in ICD-10-CM is illustrated in Figure 8.6.

For example, if a patient is poisoned by penicillin by taking an overdose accidentally, the encounter would be coded using the ICD-10-CM Table of Drugs and Chemicals in category T36.0x1. If the patient takes the correct prescribed dosage of penicillin and has an adverse reaction, the encounter is still reported using T36.0x1 because in ICD-10-CM both are considered a poisoning.

FIGURE 8.6 Excerpt From ICD-10-CM Table of Drugs and Chemicals

Substance	Poisoning, Accidental (unintentional)	Poisoning, Intentional (self-harm)	Poisoning Assault	Poisoning Undetermined	Adverse effect	Underdosing
Pempidine	T44.2x1	T44.2x2	T44.2x3	T44.2x4	T44.2x5	T44.2x6
Penamecillin	T36.0x1	T36.0x2	T36.0x3	T36.0x4	T36.0x5	T44.2x6
Penbutolol	T44.7x1	T44.7x2	T44.7x3	T44.7x4	T44.7x5	T44.7x6
Penethamate	T36.0x1	T36.0x2	T36.0x3	T36.0x4	T36.0x5	T36.0x6
Penfluridol	T43.591	T43.592	T43.593	T43.594	T43.595	T43.596
Penflutizide	T50.2x1	T50.2x2	T50.2x3	T50.2x4	T50.2x5	T50.2x6
Pengitoxin	T46.0x1	T46.0x2	T46.0x3	T46.0x4	T46.0x5	T46.0x6
Penicillamine	T50.6x1	T50.6x2	T50.6x3	T50.6x4	T50.6x5	T50.6x6
Penicillin (any)	T36.0x1	T36.0x2	T36.0x3	T36.0x4	T36.0x5	T36.0x6
Penicillinase	T45.3x1	T45.3x2	T45.3x3	T45.3x4	T45.3x5	T45.3x6
Penicilloyl polylysine	T50.8x1	T50.8x2	T50.8x3	T50.8x4	T50.8x5	T50.8x6
Penimepicycline	T36.4x1	T36.4x2	T36.4x3	T36.4x4	T36.4x5	T36.4x6
Pentachloroethane	T53.6x1	T53.6x2	T53.6x3	T53.6x4	–	–
Pentachloronaphthalene	T53.7x1	T53.7x2	T53.7x3	T53.7x4	–	–
Pentachlorophenol (pesticide)	T60.3x1	T60.3x2	T60.3x3	T60.3x4	–	–
- herbicide	T60.3x1	T60.3x2	T60.3x3	T60.3x4	–	–
- insecticie	T60.1x1	T60.1x2	T60.1x3	T60.1x4	–	–
Pentaerythritol tetranirate	T46.3x1	T46.3x2	T46.3x3	T46.3x4	T46.3x5	T46.3x6
Pentaerythritol	T46.3x1	T46.3x2	T46.3x3	T46.3x4	T46.3x5	T46.3x6
- chloral	T42.6x1	T42.6x2	T42.6x3	T42.6x4	T42.6x5	T42.6x6
- tetranitrate NEC	T46.3x1	T46.3x2	T46.3x3	T46.3x4	T46.3x5	T46.3x6
Pentaerythrityl tetranitrate	T46.3x1	T46.3x2	T46.3x3	T46.3x4	T46.3x5	T46.3x6
Pentagastrin	T50.8x1	T50.8x2	T50.8x3	T50.8x4	T50.8x5	T50.8x6
Pentalin	T53.6x1	T53.6x2	T53.6x3	T53.6x4	–	–
Pentamethonium bromide	T44.2x1	T44.2x2	T44.2x3	T44.2x4	T44.2x5	T44.2x6
Pentamidine	T37.3x1	T37.3x2	T37.3x3	T37.3x4	T37.3x5	T37.3x6
Pentanol	T51.3x1	T51.3x2	T52.3x3	T51.3x4	–	–
Pentapyrrolinium (bitartrate)	T44.2x1	T44.2x2	T44.2x3	T44.2x4	T44.2x5	T44.2x6
Pentaquine	T37.2x1	T37.2x2	T37.2x3	T37.2x4	T37.2x5	T37.2x6
Pentazocine	T40.4x1	T40.4x2	T40.4x3	T40.4x3	T40.4x5	T40.4x6
Pentetrazole	T50.7x1	T50.7x2	T50.7x3	T50.7x4	T50.7x5	T50.7x6
Penthienate bromide	T44.3x1	T44.3x2	T44.3x3	T44.3x4	T44.3x5	T44.3x6
Pentifylline	T46.7x1	T46.7x2	T467x3	T46.7x4	T46.7x5	T46.7x6
Pentobarbital	T42.3x2	T42.3x2	T42.3x3	T42.3x4	T42.3x5	T42.3x6
- sodium	T42.3x2	T42.3x2	T42.3x3	T42.3x4	T42.3x5	T42.3x6

ICD-10-CM Table of Drugs and Chemicals; 2009

Fifth Character X Place Holder

When reviewing Figure 8.6, notice that the fifth character x is part of many of these codes. The fifth character x in many of the codes in categories T36 through T65 is a dummy placeholder to allow for possible future expansion. The x must remain in the code, and no other character should be used in its place.

Sequencing of Poisonings, Toxic Effects, Adverse Effects, and Underdosing

When poisoning is sequenced, code first from category T36 through T50. The nature of the poisoning, according to the code that specifies the nature of the poisoning, toxic effect, or adverse effect, is reported secondarily (patient's condition).

Poisonings, Toxic Effects, Adverse Effects, and Underdosing in a Pregnant Patient

DOCUMENTATION TIP

Use a code from the *Undetermined* column only when the intent of the poisoning or toxic effect cannot be determined.

Codes from Chapter 15 – Pregnancy, Childbirth, and the Puerperium are always sequenced first on a medical record. A code from subcategory O9A.21 (Injury, poisoning and certain other consequences of external causes complicating pregnancy, childbirth, and the puerperium) should be sequenced first, followed by the appropriate poisoning, toxic effect, adverse effect, or underdosing code and the additional code(s) that specify the nature of the poisoning, toxic effect, adverse effect, or underdosing.

Other T Codes that Include the External Cause

Certain other T codes are combination codes that include the external cause. For example, the codes in categories T15 through T19 (Effects of foreign body entering through natural orifice) identify the foreign body as well as the resulting injury. The intent for these codes is accidental. No secondary external-cause code is needed.

T15 identifies a foreign body on the external eye. Codes from T15 through T19 require extension codes to identify whether the visit is the initial encounter, a subsequent encounter, or an encounter to address a sequela of the injury. These codes are generally the same as comparable codes in ICD-9-CM.

For example, a construction worker was cutting metal, and a metal shaving penetrated the cornea of the right eye. The patient went to an ophthalmologist, who removed the foreign body and patched the eye. Because this was the initial injury, the fifth digit extension is *a* for the initial encounter. The encounter is reported as T15.01A, Foreign body in cornea, right eye.

For category T71 (Asphyxiation) in addition to the external cause and the resulting injury, the intent is included as the final character. The final characters are as follows:

1   Accidental (unintentional)

2   Intentional self-harm

3   Assault

4   Undetermined.

The ICD-10-CM categories are very similar to the ICD-9-CM codes for the same conditions, but ICD-10-CM provides added specificity. In ICD-9-CM, the code for asphyxiation and strangulation is 994.7. In ICD-10-CM, asphyxiation has three codes in T71-:

- T71.1-   Asphyxiation due to mechanical threat to breathing
- T71.2-   Asphyxiation due to systemic oxygen deficiency due to low oxygen content in ambient air
- T71.9-   Asphyxiation due to unspecified cause.

When no intent is indicated, the default is *accidental. Undetermined intent* is used only when there is specific documentation in the medical record that the intent of the poisoning or toxic effect cannot be determined.

For example, a seven-year-old patient was playing in an old refrigerator and closed the door, causing asphyxiation. The mother found the child, and he was taken to an emergency department. The diagnosis code is reported as T71.231, Asphyxiation due to being trapped in a (discarded) refrigerator, accidental. The sixth character *1* identifies the asphyxiation as accidental.

Adult and Child Abuse, Neglect, and Other Maltreatment

ICD-10-CM has two categories for abuse and neglect: T74 (Adult and child abuse, neglect, and other maltreatment, confirmed) and T76 (Adult and child abuse, neglect, and other maltreatment, suspected). The principal/first listed diagnosis is reported with T74 or T76, followed by the mental health or injury code(s). If abuse or neglect is confirmed in the medical record, the encounter is coded as confirmed. If the documentation indicates suspected, it is coded as suspected. If the neglect, abuse, or mistreatment is ruled out, code Z04.7- is reported.

Z04.71   Encounter for examination and observation following alleged physical abuse

Z04.72   Encounter for examination and observation following alleged child physical abuse

A code from T76 should not be reported.

Use of an External-Cause Code with an Abuse or Neglect Code

When a confirmed case of physical abuse is documented, external-cause codes are reported. A code for the external cause Y08- should be reported in addition to the place of occurrence (Y92-), if known. These codes should be reported as additional diagnoses, following the injury code for any physical injuries treated. In addition, a perpetrator code (Y07) should be added when the perpetrator of the abuse is known.

Review the following comparison between ICD-9-CM and ICD-10-CM in the following example and in Figure 8.7: A ten-year-old child spilled her milk at the kitchen table during breakfast, and her father poured scalding hot water on her right hand as punishment, causing a second degree burn on the child's hand, which needed treatment. The patient was taken to the emergency department of the local hospital by her mother, and social services was contacted by a concerned physician.

FIGURE 8.7 Comparison Between ICD-9-CM and ICD-10-CM for Coding of Child Abuse

ICD-9-CM		ICD-10-CM	
944.20	Second degree burn of the hand, unspecified site	T23.201A	Burn of second degree of right hand, unspecified site
E968.3	Assault by hot liquid	Y08.89A	Assault by other specified means
E849.0	Place of occurrence, home	Y92.010	Kitchen of single-family (private) house as the place of occurrence of the external cause
		Y07.11	Biological father as perpetrator of maltreatment and neglect

---

Abuse and Other Maltreatment in a Pregnant Patient

Codes from Chapter 15: Pregnancy, Childbirth, and the Puerperium are always sequenced first on a medical record. A code(s) from subcategories O9A.3- (Physical abuse complicating pregnancy, childbirth, and the puerperium), O9A.4- (Sexual abuse complicating pregnancy, childbirth, and the puerperium), and O9A.5- (Psychological abuse complicating pregnancy, childbirth, and the puerperium) should be sequenced first, followed by any accompanying mental health or injury codes. No code from category T74 or T76 is needed.

Complication Codes that Include the External Cause

In block T80 through T88 (Complications of surgical and medical care, not elsewhere classified), the user is advised to use an additional external-cause code to identify the device and circumstances involved in the procedure that resulted in complications. The codes are very similar to codes for the same circumstances in ICD-9-CM but offer greater specificity. No external-cause code indicating the type of procedure is necessary with a code from T81.5. Review Figure 8.8, which is an example of T81-.

**FIGURE 8.8 Excerpt From ICD-10-CM
Tabular List, T81.5**

T81.5   Complications of foreign body accidentally left in body following procedure

   T81.50   Unspecified complication of foreign body accidentally left in body
             following procedure

   T81.51   Adhesions due to foreign body accidentally left in body following
             procedure

   T81.52   Obstruction due to foreign body accidentally left in body follow-
             ing procedure

   T81.53   Perforation due to foreign body accidentally left in body following
             procedure

   T81.59   Other complications of foreign body accidentally left in body fol-
             lowing procedure

Mechanical Complications

A mechanical complication of a medical device, implant, or graft is defined as one of the following:

1   Mechanical breakdown

2   Displacement or malposition

3   Leakage

4   Obstruction

5   Perforation

6   Protrusion.

If a repair of a medical device, implant, or graft is done to correct one of these complications, a mechanical complication code should be assigned.

The number of codes available to code mechanical complications has increased dramatically in ICD-10-CM compared to that in ICD-9-CM. For example, the ICD-9-CM code for mechanical complications resulting from a breast prosthesis has only one code, 996.54. In ICD-10-CM, a mechanical complication of a breast prosthesis is based on whether the complication is a breakdown of the breast prosthesis, displacement of the breast prosthesis, leakage, or other complication. Review Figure 8.9 as the example.

**FIGURE 8.9 Excerpt From ICD-10-CM
Tabular List, T85.4**

T85.4   Mechanical complication of breast prosthesis and implant

   T85.41   Breakdown (mechanical) of breast prosthesis and implant

   T85.42   Displacement of breast prosthesis and implant

   T85.43   Leakage of breast prosthesis and implant

   T85.49   Other mechanical complication of breast prosthesis and implant

Organ Transplant Complications

The remaining T codes are used to code complications of transplanted organs and tissue, complications peculiar to reattachment and amputation, and other complications of surgical and medical care, not elsewhere classified. Organ transplant rejection, failure, and infection are complications. Category T86 (Complications of transplanted organs and tissue) has codes for these specified types of complications. If a physician documents that another problem a patient is experiencing is associated with a transplanted organ, it should also be coded as a complication.

Chapter 20 – External Causes of Morbidity

External-cause codes for injuries and other health conditions provide data for research and prevention strategies. These codes capture the cause of the injury or health condition and have been further expanded in ICD-10-CM compared to ICD-9-CM. The external-cause codes are similar to the E codes in ICD-9-CM, which identify the intent of the circumstance, including:

- unintentional (accidental);
- intentional (self-harm or assault);
- the place where the event occurred; and
- the activity of the patient at the time of the event.

External-cause codes are never to be recorded as a principal/first listed diagnosis as with the E codes in ICD-9-CM. These codes can be used in any health care setting. They are useful in identifying the external source of an injury or disease. As with the E codes in ICD-9-CM, as many external-cause codes as necessary to fully explain each cause may be used.

Sequencing of multiple external-cause codes is based on the sequence of events leading to the injury. If only one external-cause code can be recorded, assign the code that relates to the principal/first listed diagnosis.

External-cause code categories include the following:

- V00–V58   Accidents
- V00   Transport accidents
- V00–V09   Pedestrian injured in transport accident
- V10–V19   Pedal cyclist injured in transport accident
- V20–V29   Motorcycle rider injured in transport accident
- V30–V39   Occupant of three-wheeled motor vehicle injured in transport accident
- V40–V49   Car occupant injured in transport accident
- V50–V59   Occupant of pick-up truck or van injured in transport accident
- V60–V69   Occupant of heavy transport vehicle injured in transport accident
- V70–V79   Bus occupant injured in transport accident
- V80–V89   Other land transport accidents
- V90–V94   Water transport accidents

- V95–V97   Air and space transport accidents
- V98–V99   Other and unspecified transport accidents
- W00–X58   Other external causes of accidental injury
- W00–W19   Slipping, tripping, stumbling, and falls
- W20–W49   Exposure to inanimate mechanical forces
- W50–W64   Exposure to animate mechanical forces
- W65–W74   Accidental nontransport drowning and submersion
- W85–W99   Exposure to electric current, radiation, and extreme ambient air temperature and pressure
- X00–X08   Exposure to smoke, fire, and flames
- X10–X19   Contact with heat and hot substances
- X30–X39   Exposure to forces of nature
- X52, X58   Accidental exposure to other specified factors
- X71–X83   Intentional self-harm
- X92–Y08   Assault
- Y21–Y33   Event of undetermined intent
- Y35–Y38   Legal intervention, operations of war, military operations, and terrorism
- Y62–Y84   Complications of medical and surgical care
- Y62–Y69   Misadventures to patients during surgical and medical care
- Y70–Y82   Medical devices associated with adverse incidents in diagnostic and therapeutic use
- Y83–Y84   Surgical and other medical procedures as the cause of abnormal reaction of the patient or of later complication, without mention of misadventure at the time of the procedure
- Y90–Y99   Supplementary factors related to causes of morbidity classified elsewhere.

Some of the external-cause codes are combination codes that identify sequential events that result in an injury, such as a fall that results in striking against an object. The injury may be due to either event or both. The combination external-cause code used should correspond to the sequence of events, regardless of which caused the most serious injury. External-cause codes for child and adult abuse take sequencing priority over all other external-cause codes.

Activity Codes

New to ICD-10-CM are activity codes. Activity codes are reported with category Y93- as secondary codes to identify the activity at the time of injury. Use an activity code only one time per patient encounter. This code should be reported only for the initial encounter for treatment and not be used for subsequent care. Always use an activity code along with a place of occurrence code. Activity codes have a seventh character extension for reporting the type of activity. The seventh character extensions for Y93- are the following:

1   Non-work–related activity

2   Work-related activity done for income

3   Student activity

4   Activity performed while a student, not for income

5   Military activity.

If a patient is a student but performing an activity for income, report the seventh character 2 for the work-related activity. If the activity of the patient is not documented, report Y93.9 for unspecified activity.

Place of Occurrence

In ICD-9-CM, place of occurrence codes are classified as 849.4. The fourth digit identifies the location of the occurrence. In ICD-10-CM, codes from category Y92 (Place of occurrence of the external cause) are secondary codes for use with other external-cause codes to identify the location of the patient at the time of injury. In ICD-9-CM, the place of occurrence codes are more limiting than in ICD-10-CM. A place of occurrence code is used only once, at the initial encounter for treatment. A place of occurrence code should be used in conjunction with an activity code, Y93-. Use place of occurrence code Y92.9 if the place is not stated or is not applicable. Place of occurrence codes are not necessary with poisonings, toxic effects, adverse effects, or underdosing codes. No extensions are used for Y92-. No seventh character is used for place of occurrence codes.

For example, while on a skiing vacation in Aspen, a patient fell and suffered a stress fracture of the right femur. The codes are as follows:

Principal/first listed diagnosis–M84.351A	Stress fracture, right femur
Secondary Diagnosis–V00.32	Snow-ski accident-fall from snow skis
Activity–Y93.29	Other individual sport
Place of occurrence–Y92.39	Other specified sports and athletic area as the place of occurrence of the external cause

When the stress fracture is coded, the seventh character *A* identifies the initial treatment. Also, because this was a non-work or student activity, the activity code requires a 1 extension (non-work related activity). The place of occurrence code(s) should only be reported at the initial encounter for treatment.

The place of occurrence (Y92-) and activity codes (Y93-) are sequenced after the main external-cause code. Regardless of the number of external-cause codes assigned, there should be only one place of occurrence code and one activity code assigned to a record. The place of occurrence codes have been expanded significantly in ICD-10-CM compared to ICD-9-CM.

Sequencing Priority

External-cause codes have a specific sequencing priority, as in ICD-9-CM:

- Terrorism takes sequencing priority over all other external-cause codes.
  Exception: child and adult abuse

- Cataclysmic events take sequencing priority over all other external-cause codes.
  Exception: child and adult abuse and terrorism

- Transport accidents take sequencing priority over all other external-cause codes.
  Exception: cataclysmic events, child and adult abuse, and terrorism

Selection of the appropriate external-cause code is guided by the Index to External Causes, a separate index in ICD-10-CM, and by the instructional notes in Chapter 20. The code indicated in the Index for the main term is verified in the Tabular List of Chapter 20. The conventions and rules for the classification also apply. There are also sections for legal interventions, operations of war, military operations, terrorism, complications of medical and surgical care, and supplemental factors related to causes of morbidity classified elsewhere.

External Cause Code Extensions

Codes from categories V00 through Y35 require an extension to indicate whether the encounter is the initial encounter for treatment, a subsequent encounter for treatment, or the sequela of an event.

The extensions for these categories are as follows:

A Initial encounter
D Subsequent encounter
S Sequela.

These extensions match the extensions for the nonfracture T codes that have extensions. An external-cause code may be used for every health care encounter for the duration of treatment of an illness or injury.

Different extensions are needed for Y93, Activity code. No extensions are required for categories Y62 through Y84 (Complications of medical and surgical care).

Unintentional (Accidental) Injuries

The default for external cause is *unintentional*. If there is no documentation in the medical record as to the intent of an injury, it should be assigned an *unintentional intent* external-cause code.

Transport Accidents

The type of vehicle in which a patient is an occupant is identified in the first two characters, because it is seen as the most important factor to identify for prevention purposes. A transport accident is one in which the vehicle involved is moving or running or in use for transport purposes at the time of the accident. When accidents involving more than one kind of transport are recorded, the following order of precedence should be used:

- V95–V97   Aircraft and spacecraft
- V90–V94   Watercraft
- V00–V89, V98–V99   Other modes of transport.

When transport accident descriptions do not specify the victim as being a vehicle occupant, and the victim is described by terms such as *crushed*, *dragged*, *hit*, or *run over*, classify the victim as a pedestrian. If no documentation is available as to whether the victim was the driver or occupant of a vehicle, classify the victim as an occupant. Use additional external-cause codes with a transport accident code to identify:

- the use of a cell phone or other electronic equipment contributing to the accident (Y93.c2);
- whether an airbag contributed to any injury (W22.1); and
- the type of street or road where the accident occurred, if known, (Y92.4-).

Falls

From ICD-9-CM, subcategory E883.0 (Accident from diving or jumping into water [swimming pool]) has been expanded in ICD-10-CM. Categories W00 through W19 (Falls) include the main fall codes in Chapter 20 (see Figure 8.10). These codes are for standard types of falls, such as falls on ice and snow or falling from stairs or off a ladder. There are other fall codes in Chapter 20 for falls associated with other causes, such as the following:

- Fires
- Watercraft accidents
- Pedestrian
- Conveyance accidents
- Subsequent striking against objects.

**FIGURE 8.10 Excerpt From ICD-10-CM
Tabular List, W16**

W16   Fall, jump or diving into water
The following seventh character extensions are to be added to each code
from category W16:
A initial encounter
D subsequent encounter
S sequelae

W16.0   Fall into swimming pool
W16.01   Fall into swimming pool striking water surface
W16.011   Fall into swimming pool striking water sur-
face causing drowning and submersion
W16.012   Fall into swimming pool striking water sur-
face causing other injury

W16.02   Fall into swimming pool striking bottom
W16.021   Fall into swimming pool striking bottom causing drowning and submersion
W16.022   Fall into swimming pool striking bottom causing other injury

W16.03   Fall into swimming pool striking wall
W16.031   Fall into swimming pool striking wall causing
drowning and submersion
W16.032   Fall into swimming pool striking wall causing
other injury

For example, a four-year-old male at a public pool tripped on the concrete and
fell into the water, hitting his head on the wall of the pool, which resulted in a
contusion of the head. The mother took the child to an emergency department
for care. Codes are reported in the following manner, using the guideline for
external causes:

Principal/first listed diagnosis–S00.93A	Contusion of unspecified part of head (illness or injury code)
External cause–W16.032	Fall into swimming pool, striking wall, causing other injury
Place of occurrence–Y92.34	Swimming pool (public) as the place of occurrence of the external cause
Activity–Y93.11	Swimming (seventh character 1 for non-work–related activity)

Assault

An assault is an intentional infliction of an injury to another person with intent
to injure or kill. Assault codes are classified X92 through Y08. They identify the

external cause of injury. Other codes are available for terrorism, military operations, operations of war, and legal interventions. Assault codes are not used in these circumstances.

Undetermined Intent

The default for injuries when the documentation does not indicate intent is *unintentional*. Codes from categories Y20 through Y33 (Events of undetermined intent) are used only when the documentation specifically states that the intent cannot be determined.

Legal Interventions

In ICD-9-CM, codes for legal interventions are E codes for classification by injury. The codes from category Y35 (Legal intervention) are used with any injury documented as sustained as a result of an encounter with any law enforcement official serving in any capacity at the time of the encounter, whether the official is on or off duty. The sixth character for the legal intervention codes identifies the victim, a law enforcement official, a bystander, or the suspect of a crime.

The seventh character extensions for Y35 are the same as for the majority of categories, to identify the encounter as for initial, subsequent, or sequela treatment as in the following list:

A Initial encounter
D Subsequent encounter
S Sequela.

Review the following example of legal intervention codes:
- Y35.00   Legal intervention involving unspecified firearm discharge
               Legal intervention involving gunshot wound
               Legal intervention involving a shot NOS
- Y35.001   Legal intervention involving unspecified firearm discharge, law enforcement official injured
- Y35.002   Legal intervention involving unspecified firearm discharge, bystander injured.
- Y93.003   Legal intervention involving unspecified firearm discharge, suspect injured.

The condition of the patient should be reported as the principal/first listed diagnosis, and the cause (Legal intervention) should be reported as a secondary diagnosis.

Operations of War/Military Operations

Category Y36 (Operations of war) is limited to classifying injuries sustained during a time of declared war, which are directly caused by the war. The code Y37 (Military operations) is used to classify injuries to military and civilian personnel occurring during peacetime on military property or during routine military exercises or operations. The extensions for Y36 and Y37 are the same as for the majority of categories for the initial encounter (A), subsequent encounter (D), and sequela (S).

Transport accidents during peacetime involving military vehicles that are off military property are included with transport accidents, not in Y36 or Y37.

Chapter 21 – Factors Influencing Health Status and Contact with Health Services

When codes in ICD-10-CM Chapter 21 are compared with V codes from the ICD-9-CM Supplementary Classification of Factors Influencing Health Status and Contact with Health Services (V01-V89), it is evident that codes have been added, deleted, combined, or moved from one section or chapter to another in ICD-10-CM.

Codes in Chapter 21 – Factors Influencing Health Status and Contact With Health Services (Z codes) are provided to deal with occasions when circumstances other than a disease or injury classifiable to the other chapters of ICD-10-CM are recorded as a reason for encounters with a health care provider. There are four primary circumstances for the use of Z codes:

1   When a person who is not currently sick has a health care encounter for some specific reason

2   When a person with a resolving disease or injury or a chronic, long-term condition requiring continuous care has a health care encounter for specific aftercare of that disease or injury

3   When circumstances or problems influence a person's health status but are not in themselves a current illness or injury

4   For newborns, to indicate birth status.

> **GUIDELINE TIP**
>
> A diagnosis/symptom code, not a Z code, should be used whenever a current, acute condition is being treated or a sign or symptom is being studied.

Z codes are used in both the inpatient and outpatient setting but are generally used more often in the outpatient setting. They may be used as either principal/first listed codes or as secondary codes, depending on the circumstances of the encounter. Certain Z codes may be first listed only, others secondary only. Documentation in the medical record must support the Z code assigned for the patient encounter.

General and Administrative Examinations

General and administrative examinations are reported for encounters for routine examinations. The codes from these categories are first listed codes. They are not for use if the examination is for diagnosis of a suspected condition or for treatment purposes. In such cases, a confirmed diagnosis, sign, or symptom code should be used. Codes in the category range from Z00 through Z13. For example, an encounter for a well-child check is reported in ICD-9-CM with code V20.2, but in ICD-10-CM there are two code options for this classification—Z00.121 and Z00.129. Review Figure 8.11.

> ### FIGURE 8.11 Excerpt From ICD-10-CM Tabular List, Z00.1
>
> Z00.121 Encounter for routine child health examination with abnormal findings
> > Use an additional code to identify any abnormal findings
>
> > Z00.129 Encounter for routine child health examination without abnormal findings
> > > Encounter for routine child health examination NOS
> > Z00.12   Encounter for routine child health examination
> > > Encounter for development testing of infant or child
> > > > Excludes 1: health supervision of foundling or other healthy infant or child (Z76.1-Z76.2)

The instructional notes in Z00.121 indicate that if abnormal findings are discovered during a routine examination, the abnormal findings are reported as secondary codes. There is an instructional note, *Excludes1*, to report health supervision with Z76.1 through Z76.2. Code Z76.1 is for health supervision and care of a foundling, and Z76.2 is reported for other health supervision of a healthy infant or child. This category is used for the following:

- Encounter for medical or nursing care or supervision of healthy infant under circumstances such as adverse socioeconomic conditions at home
- Encounter for medical or nursing care or supervision of healthy infant under circumstances such as awaiting foster or adoptive placement
- Encounter for medical or nursing care or supervision of healthy infant under circumstances such as maternal illness
- Encounter for medical or nursing care or supervision of healthy infant under circumstances such as number of children at home preventing or interfering with normal care.

Category Z00 (Encounter for general examination without complaint, suspected or reported diagnosis) and category Z01 (Encounter for other special examination without complaint or suspected or reported diagnosis) include subcategories for general medical examinations including eye, ear, and dental examinations, general laboratory and radiology examinations, and routine child health examinations as well as encounters for examinations for potential organ donors and controls for participants in clinical trials.

Category Z02 (Encounter for administrative examinations) includes codes for such things as pre-employment physicals. The final character of the general health examination codes distinguishes between *without abnormal findings* and *with abnormal findings*. For these encounters, if an abnormal condition is discovered, the code for *with abnormal findings* should be used. A secondary code for the specific abnormal finding should be used.

For example, a 30-year-old, healthy male with no complaints went to his internist for his annual physical examination. The physician counseled the patient on diet and exercise and diagnosed the patient as a healthy male with no significant findings. The codes are as follows:

Principal/first listed diagnosis–Z00.00   Encounter for general adult
medical examination without
abnormal findings

The preoperative examination codes are reported with Z01.81 through Z01.818 and are used for surgical clearance when no other treatment is provided. Pre-existing and chronic conditions may also be assigned with codes from Z00.- through Z02.-, as long as the examination does not focus on them.

For example, a patient with a history of heart disease who was scheduled for hip surgery was sent to a cardiologist for preoperative clearance. Review the comparison between ICD-9-CM and ICD-10-CM in Figure 8.12.

FIGURE 8.12 Comparison Between ICD-9-CM and ICD-10-CM for Coding of Preoperative Cardiovascular Examination

ICD-9-CM		ICD-10-CM	
V72.81	Preoperative cardiovascular examinations	Z01.810	Encounter for preprocedural cardiovascular examination

Observation

There are two observation categories in ICD-10-CM:
- Z03   Encounter for medical observation for suspected diseases and conditions
- Z04   Encounter for observation for other reasons.

An observation encounter is coded when a person without a diagnosis is suspected of having an abnormal condition following an accident or incident that might result in a health problem, but without signs or symptoms, that, after examination and observation, is ruled out. These codes are used in very limited circumstances when a person is being observed for a suspected condition that is found not to exist. The fact that the patient may be scheduled for a return encounter following the initial observation encounter does not limit the use of an observation code.

For example, a six-year-old patient was transported by ambulance to an emergency department following a car accident. The mother was driving on an icy road, and the minivan she was driving flipped on its top. After doing an examination in which no significant injuries were identified, the physician decided to observe the child for a few hours before releasing her from the emergency department. The first listed diagnosis is Z04.1, Encounter for examination and observation following transport accident.

Pre-existing and chronic conditions may also be assigned with codes from Z03 through Z04, as long as they are not associated with the suspected condition being observed.

GUIDELINE TIP

Do not use an observation code for a patient with any illness, injury, or signs and symptoms. The illness, injury, signs, or symptoms should be coded with the corresponding external-cause code.

Follow-Up

The follow-up codes are used to describe continuing patient encounters following completed treatment of a disease, condition, or injury. Follow-up care should not be confused with aftercare that explains current treatment for a healing or long-term condition.

A patient who is being followed for a history of a condition that has healed, or resolved condition, but still requires repeated visits will be reported with an ICD-10-CM follow-up code along with the history code for the condition previously treated. For instance, a patient who had cancer will require long-term follow-up care, and a history code is reported after the cancer has been eradicated. If the condition is still present or reoccurs, the follow-up visit code should be reported in addition to the condition diagnosed during the visit.

Codes used in this category include the following:

- Z08   Encounter for follow-up examination after completed treatment for malignant neoplasm
- Z09   Encounter for follow-up examination after completed treatment for conditions other than malignant neoplasm.

When a Z08 code is reported, it is necessary to assign the appropriate secondary code from category Z85 (Personal history of primary and secondary malignant neoplasm). Review the following example: A 45-year-old female patient was seen by the oncologist in follow-up after breast cancer treatment two years earlier. There was no sign of recurrence.

Review the comparison between ICD-9-CM and ICD-10-CM in Figure 8.13.

FIGURE 8.13 Comparison Between ICD-9-CM and ICD-10-CM for Coding of Follow-Up Encounter After Treatment for Neoplasm

ICD-9-CM		ICD-10-CM	
V10.3	History of malignant neoplasm of the breast	Z08	Encounter for follow-up examination after completed treatment for malignant neoplasm
		Z85.3	Personal history of primary malignant neoplasm of breast

---

Screenings

Screening is the testing for disease or disease precursors in seemingly healthy individuals so that early detection and treatment can be provided for those who test positive for the disease. The testing of a person to rule out or confirm a suspected diagnosis because the patient has some sign or symptom is a diagnostic test, not a screening. For these cases, the code for the sign or symptom, not the screening code, is used to explain the test.

A screening code may be a first listed code if the reason for the encounter is specifically the screening. The code may also be used as an additional code if the screening is done during an encounter for other health reasons.

A screening code is not necessary if the screening is inherent to a routine examination, such as a Pap smear done during a routine pelvic examination.

If a condition is discovered during a screening, the screening code should still be used, followed by the code for the condition that is discovered. ICD-10-CM category codes Z11 through Z13 are used to report encounters for specific screening examinations.

The screening categories are as follows:

- Z11   Encounter for screening for infectious and parasitic diseases
- Z12   Encounter for screening for malignant neoplasms
- Z13   Encounter for screening for other diseases and disorders.

For example, a screening mammogram was performed on a 50-year-old woman with no personal or family history of cancer. The encounter is reported as Z12.31, Encounter for screening mammogram for malignant neoplasm of breast.

Contact/Exposure

ICD-10-CM category codes Z20 through Z28 are assigned to the records of persons who have been diagnosed as having communicable diseases that pose potential public health hazards. These codes are used for patients who do not have any signs or symptoms of a disease but have been exposed either by close personal contact or where an epidemic has erupted. These codes may be reported as the principal/first listed diagnosis to explain the patient encounter or testing performed or may be used as a secondary diagnosis to report the potential risk.

For example, a 15-year-old female was playing with a puppy at a neighbor's home. It was discovered two days later that the puppy had rabies. The patient was taken to her family physician by her mother for evaluation of the situation and determination of treatment options. The principal/first listed diagnosis is Z20.3, Contact with and exposure to rabies. In ICD-9-CM, this encounter for the exposure to rabies would be reported with V01.5.

Status

Status codes indicate that a patient is either a carrier of a disease or has the sequela or residual of a past disease or condition. This includes such things as the use of a prosthetic or mechanical device. A status code is informative because the status may affect any current treatment and its outcome. A status code is distinct from a history code. A history code indicates that the patient no longer has a condition. Codes in the category are used for situations such as identifying long-term care of drug therapy, identifying a pregnant patient whose condition is incidental to patient visits for treatment, and for a patient who is HIV positive with no symptoms.

When a patient has a drug allergy, codes from this category should be added to the record at every encounter, because this condition is chronic and is typically a lifelong condition. This subcategory includes allergies to foods, insects, and other nonmedicinal substances, such as latex.

Review some of the status Z categories/subcategory/codes in ICD-10-CM:

- Z14   Genetic carrier
- Z15   Genetic susceptibility to disease
- Z16   Infection with drug-resistant microorganism
- Z17   Estrogen receptor status
- Z20   Contact with and (suspected) exposure to communicable diseases
- Z21   Asymptomatic human immunodeficiency virus [HIV] infection status
- Z22   Carrier of infectious disease
- Z33.–   Pregnant state
- Z66   Do not resuscitate
- Z67   Blood type.

For example, a 28-year-old pregnant patient visited her obstetrician with a complaint of congestion and cough. The physician diagnosed the patient with influenza and an acute respiratory infection. Review the comparison between ICD-9-CM and ICD-10-CM in Figure 8.14.

FIGURE 8.14 Comparison Between ICD-9-CM and ICD-10-CM for Coding of Influenza in a Pregnant Patient

ICD-9-CM		ICD-10-CM	
487.1	Influenza with acute respiratory infection	J10.1	Influenza due to other influenza virus with respiratory manifestations
V22.2	Pregnancy state, incidental	Z33.1	Pregnancy state, incidental

Categories Z89 through Z99 are for use only if there is no complication or malfunction of the organ or tissue replaced, of the amputation site, or the equipment on which the patient is dependent. These are always secondary codes.

These code categories include the following:

- Z89   Acquired absence of limb
- Z90   Acquired absence of organs, not elsewhere classified
- Z91.0   Allergy status, other than to drugs and biological substances
- Z93   Artificial opening status
- Z94   Transplanted organ and tissue status

- Z95   Presence of cardiac and vascular implants and grafts
- Z96   Presence of other functional implants
- Z97   Presence of other devices
- Z98   Other postsurgical states
- Z99   Dependence on enabling machines and devices, not elsewhere classified.

Encounter for Immunization/Immunization Not Carried Out

Code Z23 (Encounter for immunization) is used to indicate that a patient is being seen to receive a prophylactic inoculation against a disease. The injection itself must be indicated with a procedure code. This code may be used as a secondary code if the inoculation is given as a part of preventive health care, such as a well-baby visit. Instructional notes in the beginning of the category instruct the user to report the routine childhood examination as the primary/first listed diagnosis. Immunizations against many communicable diseases are required in most states for admission to school or for employment. For persons who choose not to receive an immunization for personal or health reasons, a code from category Z28 (Immunization not carried out) should be used to identify the reason a required immunization was not given.

Encounters for Health Services Related to Reproduction

The categories/codes related to reproduction include the following:
- Z30   Encounter for contraceptive management
- Z31   Encounter for procreative management
- Z32   Encounter for pregnancy test and instruction
- Z33.1   Pregnancy state, incidental
- Z33.2   Encounter for elective termination of pregnancy
- Z34   Encounter for supervision of normal pregnancy
- Z36   Encounter for antenatal screening of mother
- Z37   Outcome of delivery
- Z38   Liveborn infant according to place of birth and type of delivery
- Z39   Encounter for maternal postpartum care and examination.

These encounter codes identify the reason for the visit. Any procedures performed must be identified with a procedure code from the appropriate procedure classification.

Aftercare

Aftercare visit codes, with category titles such as *fitting and adjustment*, and *attention to artificial openings*, cover situations in which the initial treatment of a disease or injury has been performed, and the patient requires continuing care during the healing or recovery phase or for the long-term consequences of an illness. The aftercare Z codes should not be used if treatment is directed at a current disease or injury. The disease or injury code should be used in such cases. An aftercare code may also be used as a secondary code, when some type of aftercare is provided in addition to another reason for an encounter, and no diagnosis code is applicable.

Certain aftercare codes need a secondary diagnosis code to describe the resolving condition or sequela. For others, the condition is inherent in the code title. Aftercare codes are not used for mechanical complications or malfunctioning of a device.

The aftercare categories are as follows:
- Z43   Encounter for attention to artificial openings
- Z44   Encounter for fitting and adjustment of artificial arm
- Z45   Encounter for adjustment and management of other implanted devices
- Z46   Encounter for fitting and adjustment of other devices
- Z47   Orthopedic aftercare
- Z48   Encounter for other postprocedural care
- Z49   Encounter for care involving renal dialysis
- Z51   Encounter for other aftercare.

Encounter for Radiation Therapy and Chemotherapy

For patients whose encounter is specifically to receive radiation therapy and chemotherapy, the codes used are Z51.0 (Encounter for radiotherapy session) and Z51.11 (Encounter for chemotherapy). As in ICD-9-CM, the encounter for chemotherapy or radiation therapy is sequenced first, followed by the condition treated (neoplasm). When a patient is receiving both radiation and chemotherapy during the same encounter, both codes should be used, with either sequenced first.

History (of)

The two types of history (of) codes are as follows:
- Personal history
- Family history.

Personal history codes indicate a patient's past medical condition that no longer exists but that has the potential for recurrence and, therefore, may require continued monitoring. Personal history codes should be used in conjunction with follow-up codes to explain the condition being followed. Personal history codes are acceptable on any medical record, regardless of the reason for the encounter. A personal history of an illness or condition, even if no longer present, is important information that may alter the type of treatment given.

Family history codes are used when a patient has a family member or members with a particular disease, and, because of the family history, the patient is at a higher risk for the disease. Family history codes should be used in conjunction with screening codes to explain the need for a test or procedure, if a family history of the condition being screened for is applicable.

Review some of the history (of) codes in ICD-10-CM:

- Z76.81   Expected parents, prebirth pediatrician visit
- Z80   Family history of primary malignant neoplasm
- Z81   Family history of mental and behavioral disorders
- Z82   Family history of certain disabilities and chronic diseases (leading to disablement)
- Z83   Family history of other specific disorders
- Z84   Family history of other conditions
- Z85   Personal history of malignant neoplasms
- Z86   Personal history of certain other diseases
- Z87   Personal history of other diseases and conditions
- Z91.410   Personal history of adult physical and sexual abuse
- Z91.49   Other personal history of psychological trauma, not elsewhere classified
- Z91.5   Personal history of self-harm
- Z91.8   Other specified personal risk factors, not elsewhere classified
- Z92   Personal history of medical treatment.

For example, a patient with a family history of diabetes mellitus, who was healthy with no sign of the disease, visited her family physician for evaluation. Review the comparison between ICD-9-CM and ICD-10-CM in Figure 8.15.

FIGURE 8.15 Comparison Between ICD-9-CM and ICD-10-CM for Coding of Family History of Diabetes Mellitus

ICD-9-CM		ICD-10-CM	
V18.0	Family history of diabetes mellitus	Z83.3	Family history of diabetes mellitus

Category Z83- includes the family history of diabetes mellitus and is coded in ICD-10-CM as Z83.3, as illustrated.

Summary

Make sure that when ICD-10-CM is used, the guidelines are reviewed prior to the selection of the code. Even though ICD-10-CM is similar to ICD-9-CM, there are significant differences in the coding with additions of character extensions, which add additional specificity, and dummy characters that leave room for further expansion. The successful transition to ICD-10-CM requires a clear understanding and training on guidelines.

Resources

ICD-10-CM Official Guidelines for Coding and Reporting, 2009. Available online at ftp://ftp.cdc.gov/pub/Health_Statistics/NCHS/Publications/ICD10CM/2009/.

National Center for Health Statistics. *ICD-10-CM Tabular List.* Available online at ftp://ftp.cdc.gov/pub/Health_Statistics/NCHS/Publications/ICD10CM/2009/.

End-of-Chapter Questions

1   In the Table of Drugs and Chemicals, the poisoning codes for undetermined intent should be used only when:

_____ .

2   How are poisoning codes sequenced?

_____

3   The three common seventh character extensions are:

_____ .

_____ .

_____ .

4   How should spinal cord injuries be reported, based on the

ICD-10-CM guidelines? _____

5   Burn codes are classified by:

_____ .

_____ .

_____ .

CHAPTER 9

ICD-10-CM: Crosswalks and Mapping

OBJECTIVES

- Understand how to use mapping with the diagnosis code set General Equivalence Mappings (GEMs)
- Review examples of crosswalking and mapping using the GEMs files
- Review the flags in the International Classification of Diseases, Tenth Revision, Clinical Modification (ICD-10-CM) and the relationship to combination diagnosis codes

Introduction

This chapter will cover the mapping system using the National Center for Health Statistics (NCHS) General Equivalence Mappings (GEMs) files. Crosswalking and mapping ICD-9-CM to ICD-10-CM and ICD-10-CM back to ICD-9-CM is an important step regarding transitioning to ICD-10-CM. Coding comparisons will assist users in identifying codes for crosswalking and mapping. Mapping, which has been completed by NCHS, identifies the relationship between the ICD-9-CM code and the ICD-10-CM code. Crosswalks are practice sheets or software tools to establish the transition from ICD-9-CM to ICD-10-CM for more frequently used codes. The purpose of the GEMs files or mapping is to provide a temporary mechanism for mapping claims containing ICD-10 diagnoses to the reimbursement equivalent ICD-9-CM diagnoses so that while insurance carrier systems are undergoing conversion to the ICD-10-CM claims directly, the claims may be processed by the legacy systems. The ICD-10-CM diagnoses on the claim are mapped by the application of the Diagnosis Reimbursement Mapping into ICD-9-CM diagnoses used by the ICD-9-CM-based reimbursement system.

Mapping Using the GEMs

The GEMs were developed by NCHS and are in the public domain. They are diagnosis code reference mappings between ICD-9-CM and ICD-10-CM. The instructions and text file map ICD-9-CM to ICD-10-CM and ICD-10-CM to ICD-9-CM. This mapping system is a good tool to help practices create their own crosswalks for their most frequently used diagnosis codes.

Both ICD-9-CM and ICD-10-CM have GEMs files that facilitate linking between the ICD-9-CM and ICD-10-CM code sets. The GEMs files are not considered crosswalks; rather, they are more complex than a one-to-one crosswalk and are more useful. Essentially, they are a reference mapping system to assist the user in navigating the difficulty of translating the meaning of one code set to another.

Mapping is an attempt to find the corresponding diagnosis and the correlation between the two code sets. In ICD-9-CM, codes are three to five digits plus

V codes and E codes and number approximately 14,000 codes. In ICD-10-CM, the code structure is three to seven alphanumeric codes with approximately 68,000 codes. There is no simple map from ICD-9-CM to ICD-10-CM in the GEMs files. The GEMs have attempted to organize the differences between ICD-9-CM and ICD-10-CM. When a code is being mapped from ICD-9-CM to ICD-10-CM, there may be more than one code in ICD-10-CM that maps to ICD-9-CM.

The GEMs files are formatted as flat text files in which each file contains a list of code pairs that identify the correspondence between a source-system code and a target-system code. The code set is being mapped from the source system—the system of origin—to the destination (or target) system.

The GEMs files are in a text format. There is one GEMs file for mapping ICD-9-CM to ICD-10-CM and one file for backward mapping from ICD-10-CM to ICD-9-CM. Also included are the ICD-10-CM code descriptions in a text file. The ICD-9-CM code descriptions can be found at the Centers for Disease Control and Prevention (CDC) Web site at www.cdc.gov/nchs/icd9.htm#RTF.

To link a code in the source system to a combination of codes in the target system, the use of a scenario or choice list may be required. A scenario is a collection of codes from the target system that contain the necessary codes that will satisfy the meaning of a code in the source system. A choice list is a list of one or more codes from the target system in which one code must be chosen to satisfy the same meaning of a code from the source system.

It is important to distinguish between an entry of the single type and a single row in a combination entry to ensure that the mapping between ICD-9 and ICD-10 is appropriate and provides the desired information. The goal of the GEMs file is to find corresponding diagnosis codes, when possible, between ICD-9-CM and ICD-10-CM. In certain areas of the classification, the correlation between the two sets is close (ie, when they share the conventions of organization and formatting).

Examples and Coding Comparisons Between ICD-9-CM and ICD-10-CM

Example 1

A patient with type 1 diabetes and Kimmelstiel-Wilson disease visited an endocrinologist in follow-up for a routine three-month visit (see Figure 9.1).

FIGURE 9.1 **Comparison Between ICD-9-CM and ICD-10-CM for Coding of Diabetes**

ICD-9-CM		ICD-10-CM	
250.41	Diabetes with renal manifestations, type 1 [juvenile type], not stated as uncontrolled	E10.21	Type 1 diabetes mellitus with diabetic nephropathy
			Type 1 diabetes mellitus with Kimmelstiel-Wilson disease
581.81	Nephropathy, not otherwise specified	E08.21	Diabetes mellitus due to underlying condition with diabetic nephropathy

Example 2

A patient underwent an initial tympanoplasty (69631) without mastoidectomy in an outpatient hospital surgery department for an attic perforation of the tympanic membrane of the right ear (see Figure 9.2).

FIGURE 9.2 **Comparison Between ICD-9-CM and ICD-10-CM for Coding of Tympanic Membrane Perforation**

ICD-9-CM			ICD-10-CM		
384.2		Perforation of tympanic membrane	H72		Perforation of tympanic membrane
	384.20	Unspecified perforation of tympanic membrane		H72.0	Central perforation of tympanic membrane
	384.21	Central perforation of tympanic membrane		H72.1	Attic perforation of tympanic membrane
	384.22	Attic perforation of tympanic membrane			H72.10 Attic perforation of tympanic membrane, unspecified ear
	384.23	Other marginal perforation of tympanic membrane			H72.11 Attic perforation of tympanic membrane, right ear
	384.24	Multiple perforations of tympanic membrane			H72.12 Attic perforation of tympanic membrane, left ear
	384.25	Total perforation of tympanic membrane			H72.13 Attic perforation of tympanic membrane, bilateral
				H72.2	Other marginal perforations of tympanic membrane

ICD-10-CM is more specific in identifying the ear affected. Example 2 indicates that the procedure was performed on the right ear, which is reported with H72.11 (Attic perforation of tympanic membrane, right ear) in ICD-10-CM. When the choices for ICD-10-CM are reviewed, the most appropriate diagnosis code is 384.22 (Attic perforation of the tympanic membrane). ICD-9-CM is not as specific, as it does not identify which ear is affected.

The guidelines specific to the ICD-10-CM chapter involve complication of care within the body system chapter specific to the organs and structure of that body system. The condition or disease should be sequenced first, followed by a complication code in block H95, Intraoperative and postprocedural complications and disorders of ear and mastoid process, not elsewhere classified.

Example 3

A patient with a history of mastoidectomy underwent a revision of the mastoidectomy with apicectomy (69605) for cholesteatoma of the left middle ear and mastoid. During the procedure, the patient experienced hemorrhage of the ear and mastoid process. Review the comparison between ICD-9-CM and ICD-10-CM in Figure 9.3.

FIGURE 9.3 Comparison Between ICD-9-CM and ICD-10-CM for Coding of Cholesteatoma of Mastoid

ICD-9-CM		ICD-10-CM	
385.3	Cholesteatoma of middle ear and mastoid	H71.2	Cholesteatoma of mastoid
	385.30 Unspecified cholesteatoma		H71.20 Cholesteatoma of mastoid, unspecified ear
	385.31 Cholesteatoma of attic		H71.21 Cholesteatoma of mastoid, right ear
	385.32 Cholesteatoma of middle ear		H71.22 Cholesteatoma of mastoid, left ear
	385.33 Cholesteatoma of middle ear and mastoid		H71.23 Cholesteatoma of mastoid, bilateral
	385.35 Diffuse cholesteatosis of middle ear and mastoid	H71.3	Diffuse cholesteotosis

In ICD-10-CM, the diagnosis would be reported with code H71.22 (Cholesteatoma of mastoid, left ear) and with ICD-9-CM, 385.33 (Cholesteatoma of middle ear and mastoid). According to the ICD-10-CM guidelines, the complication is also coded. Review the options for coding intraoperative and postprocedural complications of the ear (H95.2), as shown below:

H95.2   Intraoperative hemorrhage and hematoma of ear and mastoid process complicating a procedure

> Excludes1: intraoperative hemorrhage and hematoma of ear and mastoid process due to accidental puncture or laceration during a procedure on the ear (H95.3-)

> H95.21   Intraoperative hemorrhage and hematoma of ear and mastoid process during a procedure on the ear and mastoid process

> H95.22   Intraoperative hematoma and hematoma of ear and mastoid process complicating other procedure

The most appropriate complication code in this block is H95.21, Intraoperative hematoma of the ear and mastoid process during a procedure of the ear and mastoid process. With ICD-9-CM, the complication would be reported in category 998.1-, Hemorrhage or hematoma or seroma complicating a procedure. A fifth digit is required in this category:

998.1   Hemorrhage or hematoma or seroma complicating a procedure
> 998.11   Hemorrhage complicating a procedure

Review the coding comparison between ICD-9-CM and ICD-10-CM in Figure 9.4.

FIGURE 9.4 **Comparison Between ICD-9-CM and ICD-10-CM for Coding of Cholesteatoma of Mastoid**

ICD-9-CM		ICD-10-CM	
385.33	Cholesteatoma of middle ear and mastoid	H71.22	Cholesteatoma of mastoid, left ear
998.11	Hemorrhage complicating a procedure	H95.22	Intraoperative hemorrhage and hematoma of ear and mastoid process complicating other procedure

---

Example 4

A patient who had been treated for hypertension for more than three years visited his internist for a three-month follow-up. He smoked currently but was not dependent on tobacco. His blood pressure was 150/100 mm Hg. The physician adjusted the dose of the patient's medication, reviewed previous blood pressure readings, counseled the patient regarding smoking cessation, and asked the patient to come back in two months. The documentation indicates benign hypertension without good control. Review the comparison between ICD-9-CM and ICD-10-CM in Figure 9.5.

FIGURE 9.5 Comparison Between ICD-9-CM and ICD-10-CM for Coding of Essential Hypertension

ICD-9-CM		ICD-10-CM	
401	Essential hypertension	I10	Essential (primary) hypertension
	401.0 Essential hypertension, malignant		Includes:
			high blood pressure
	401.1 Essential hypertension, benign		benign
			arterial
	401.9 Unspecified essential hypertension		essential
			malignant
			primary
			systemic in this category

In ICD-10-CM, Category I10 requires an additional code for tobacco exposure (Z72.0, Tobacco use), dependence, or use, which differs from ICD-9-CM. There is an *Excludes 2* note indicating that hypertension (I10) may be reported in addition to the following:

> Essential (primary) hypertension involving vessels of brain (I60-I69)
> Essential (primary) hypertension involving vessels of eye (H35.0)

Category H35.0 is reported for hypertensive retinopathy and may be used alone or with I10. If both codes are used, the sequencing is based on the reason for the encounter.

Example 5

A patient presented to the ophthalmologist for follow-up of hypertensive retinopathy. The physician determined that the retinopathy was a result of the patient's malignant hypertension. See Figure 9.6.

FIGURE 9.6 Comparison Between ICD-9-CM and ICD-10-CM for Coding of Hypertensive Retinopathy

ICD-9-CM		ICD-10-CM	
362.11	Hypertensive retinopathy	H35.033	Hypertensive retinopathy, bilateral
		I10	Essential (primary) hypertension

In ICD-9-CM, the hypertension is not reported. There is an instruction note with 401.x that excludes Hypertension with the eye (362.11). The *Excludes2* note allows reporting of both codes in ICD-10-CM.

Example 6

A patient was referred by his family physician to a gastroenterologist to rule out a bleeding ulcer. The physician performed a detailed history and examination, ordered diagnostic tests to rule out the suspected ulcer, and documented epigatric pain (upper abdomen), in the medical record.

In ICD-9-CM, the appropriate code is 789.06, Abdominal pain, epigastric. In ICD-10-CM, the code is R10.13, Epigastric pain.

Example 7

A physician diagnosed a patient who has rheumatoid polyneuropathy as having rheumatoid arthritis of the right ankle and foot. The condition is coded in ICD-10-CM using the combination code. Currently in ICD-9-CM, there is no combination code to fully describe the condition, and two codes must be used when this diagnosis is reported (see Figure 9.7).

FIGURE 9.7 Comparison Between ICD-9-CM and ICD-10-CM for Coding of Rheumatoid Arthritis

ICD-9-CM		ICD-10-CM	
714.0	Rheumatoid arthritis	M05.571	Rheumatoid polyneuropathy with rheumatoid arthritis of right ankle and foot
357.1	Polyneuropathy in collagen vascular disease		

In this example, a combination code is available in ICD-10-CM for reporting the condition.

Example 8

During a routine examination, a physician found a suspicious breast mass in the left breast of a female patient who had a history of breast cancer of the right breast. The physician scheduled a biopsy in the outpatient surgery department at the hospital. Because the diagnosis of a malignancy could not be confirmed at that visit, the breast mass was reported. In ICD-9-CM, the correct code is 611.72, Lump or mass in breast. Note that ICD-9-CM code V10.3 may be reported as an additional diagnosis for the history of breast cancer to further support medical necessity. In ICD-10-CM, the correct code is N63, Unspecified lump in breast; Includes: nodule(s) NOS in breast. In this example for category N63, the code is not further subdivided, so a three-digit category code is reported. An additional diagnosis of Z85.3 may also be reported for the personal history of breast cancer.

Example 9

A patient underwent removal of the upper lobe of the lung because of lung cancer after a mass was discovered during a computed tomography scan. See Figure 9.8.

FIGURE 9.8 Comparison Between ICD-9-CM and ICD-10-CM for Coding of Malignant Neoplasm of Lung

ICD-9-CM	ICD-10-CM
162 Malignant neoplasm of bronchus or lung	C34.1 Malignant neoplasm of upper lobe, bronchus or lung
162.3 Malignant neoplasm of upper lobe, bronchus, or lung	C34.10 Malignant neoplasm of upper lobe, bronchus or lung, unspecified side
	C34.11 Malignant neoplasm of upper right bronchus or lung
	C34.12 Malignant neoplasm of upper lobe, left bronchus or lung

---

The correct ICD-10-CM diagnosis code selection would be C34.10, because the side is not specified. Documentation in this example is extremely important as one can see, because the specificity in the documentation would indicate either the left or right lobe. It is important to begin encouraging physicians to document details more specifically so that the most appropriate diagnosis code can be selected. ICD-10-CM specifies the side of the bronchus or lung; ICD-9-CM does not have this level of specificity.

Combination Codes

One ICD-9-CM or ICD-10-CM code may contain more than one diagnosis. These are combination codes. A combination code can contain several types of diagnoses, as shown in the following examples:

ICD-9-CM

250.21 Diabetes with hyperosmolarity type 1 [juvenile type] not stated as uncontrolled

404.00 Hypertensive heart and chronic kidney disease without heart failure and with chronic kidney disease stage I through IV

823.02 Fracture of tibia and fibula shaft, open fibula and tibia

ICD-10-CM

R65.21   Severe sepsis with toxic shock

L97.114   Non-pressure chronic ulcer of right thigh with necrosis of bone

E08.21   Diabetes mellitus due to underlying condition with
diabetic nephropathy

There are also situations in which ICD-9-CM contains more detail in the code description than does ICD-10-CM. In some cases, a single ICD-9-CM code may be linked to more than one ICD-10-CM code or vice versa. Review the example in Figure 9.9.

FIGURE 9.9 **Comparison Between ICD-9-CM and ICD-10-CM for Coding of Primary Tuberculosis**

ICD-9-CM		ICD-10-CM	
010.00	Primary tuberculous infection, unspecified examination	A15.7	Primary respiratory tuberculosis
010.01	Primary tuberculous infection, bacteriological/histological examination not done		
010.02	Primary tuberculous infection, bacteriological/histological examination unknown (at present)		
010.03	Primary tuberculous infection, tubercle bacilli found by microscopy		
010.04	Primary tuberculous infection, tubercle bacilli found by bacterial culture		
010.05	Primary tuberculous infection, tubercle bacilli confirmed histologically		
010.06	Primary tuberculous infection, tubercle bacilli confirmed by other methods		

When a combination code in one code set corresponds to two or more diagnoses in the other code set, mapping requires simultaneous linkage to two or more codes in the other code set.

Mapping in ICD-9-CM and ICD-10-CM

Review the example of mapping from ICD-9-CM to ICD-10-CM in Figure 9.10.

FIGURE 9.10 Comparison Between ICD-9-CM and ICD-10-CM for Mapping of Histoplasma Meningitis

ICD-9-CM Source	ICD-10-CM Target
115.11 Histoplasma duboisii meningitis	B39.5 Histoplasmosis duboisii and G02 Meningitis in other infectious and parasitic diseases classified elsewhere

---

Now review backward mapping from ICD-10-CM to ICD-9-CM as shown in Figure 9.11.

FIGURE 9.11 Comparison Between ICD-10-CM and ICD-9-CM for Mapping of Atherosclerosis

ICD-9-CM Source	ICD-10-CM Target
414.02 Coronary atherosclerosis of autologous biological bypass graft and 411.1 Intermediate coronary syndrome	I25.710 Atherosclerosis of autologous vein coronary artery bypass graft(s) with unstable angina pectoris

---

The GEMs files are useful for facilitating linkage between the diagnosis code in ICD-9-CM and ICD-10-CM. Because these files are flat text files, they can be loaded into a database, such as Microsoft Access. A Microsoft Excel file could be used, but multiple files would need to be referenced simultaneously, which would make it cumbersome and tedious. Each file contains a list of code pairs. Each code pair identifies a correspondence between a code in the source file (ICD-9-CM or ICD-10-CM) and a code in the target system. The first step would be to perform forward mapping of ICD-9-CM to ICD-10-CM and then backward mapping of ICD-10-CM to ICD-9-CM using the GEMs files. This system will need to be used to update Superbills, practice management systems, and electronic health records. Typically, vendors will perform the mapping for information technology systems, but practices that plan to use a paper Superbill will find the GEMs files useful for updating this tool. Review the example of mapping from ICD-9-CM to ICD-10-CM shown in Figure 9.12.

FIGURE 9.12 Comparison Between ICD-9-CM
and ICD-10-CM for Mapping
of Hematuria

ICD-9-CM Source			ICD-10-CM Target	
599.7	Hematuria		R31	Hematuria
	599.71	Gross hematuria	R31.0	Gross hematuria
	599.72	Microscopic hematuria	R31.1	Benign essential microscopic hematuria
	599.72	Microscopic hematuria	R31.2	Other microscopic hematuria
	599.70	Hematuria, unspecified	R31.9	Hematuria, unspecified

Notice that in this illustration, ICD-9-CM code 599.72 (Microscopic hematuria) maps to ICD-10-CM codes R31.1 and R31.2. Documentation in the medical record will be vitally important when coding with ICD-10-CM to determine the correct diagnosis code. Review the example of mapping from ICD-10-CM to ICD-9-CM (backward mapping) shown in Figure 9.13.

FIGURE 9.13 Comparison Between ICD-9-CM
and ICD-10-CM for Backward
Mapping of Severe Sepsis With Shock

ICD-9-CM Source		ICD-10-CM Target	
995.92	Severe sepsis	R65.21	Severe sepsis with septic shock
785.52	Septic shock		

In this example, ICD-10-CM describes a combination code for severe sepsis with shock, but in ICD-9-CM, a combination code does not exist for both conditions, and each condition must be reported separately.

Mapping With GEMs Files

One ICD-9-CM or ICD-10-CM code can contain more than one diagnosis. For purposes of mapping, these are called combination codes. A combination code can contain several types of diagnoses, such as a chronic condition with a manifestation; one example would be diabetes mellitus with an ophthalmic manifestation. Alternatively, a combination code can consist of two acute conditions, such as ICD-10-CM code R65.21, Severe sepsis with septic shock. A combination code may also consist of an acute condition with an external cause, such as ICD-10-CM code T58.01, Toxic effect of carbon monoxide from motor vehicle exhaust (unintentional).

When GEMs files are used, there are two files for ICD-9-CM and ICD-10-CM. Review Figure 9.14.

FIGURE 9.14 **Excerpt From GEMs Text File, ICD-10-CM to ICD-9-CM**

ICD-10-CM	ICD-9-CM	Flags Combination Entries
R6510	99593	10000
R6510	99590	10000
R6511	99594	00000
R6520	99592	10000
R6521	99592	10111
R6521	78552	10112

Notice that the ICD-9-CM and ICD-10-CM codes do not have periods between the additional characters in column 1 and column 2. Column 1, ICD-10-CM, is the source file, because the codes to ICD-9-CM, which is the target file, are being mapped.

Mapping occurs when a combination code in one set, such as R65.21 in ICD-10-CM, corresponds to two or more diagnoses in the other set, such as 995.92 and 785.52 in ICD-9-CM. The combination code must be linked to two or more codes in the other set. In this example, R65.21 is a combination code in ICD-10-CM linked to two ICD-9-CM codes. The term *crosswalk* is often used to reference mapping between ICD-9-CM code updates. The GEMs files are not crosswalks but reference mappings to help navigate the complexity of translating meaning from one code set to the other. An entry in GEMs identifies relationships between a code in the source system and possible equivalents in the target system.

The term *entry* in the GEMs files refers to the format of the GEM, which refers to all rows in the GEM file having the same first listed code. The term *row* in the GEM file refers to a single line in the file containing a code pair—one code from the source system and one code from the target system. There are two basic types of entries in GEMs, a single entry and a combination entry.

A single entry is an entry in the GEMs for which a code in the source system is linked to one code option in the target system. However, a single entry is not one-to-one mapping in every instance. A single entry might be linked to different code(s) in the target system.

A combination entry is an entry in the GEMs for which a code in the source system must be linked to more than one code option in the target system to be a valid entry. Severe sepsis and septic shock is a good example of a combination entry.

In the GEMs, there are flags that identify combination codes that map from the source (column 1) to the target (column 2) of the table. The approximate flag is turned on when there is **not** a code in the target system or a combination code with the same meaning. The digits applicable to the flag are as follows:

- Zero (0) The approximate flag is turned off (there is **not** an equivalent diagnosis code or combination code in the target system).
- One (1) The approximate flag is turned on (there is a linked code or combination in the target system).

The first three columns after the code descriptor are called *flags*, and the last two digits are used in combination flag entries. In the GEMs files, the flags are defined as either:

- approximate—that is, the entry is not considered equivalent (this is the first digit in the third column); or
- no map, which indicates that a code in the source system is not linked to any code in the target system.

The no map flag is used when a diagnosis cannot be identified. The digits used in the no map file are 0 and 1.

- Zero (0) indicates that there is a code that maps from the source code to the target code, either a single code or combination diagnosis code. A flag does not apply and the flag is turned off.
- One (1) indicates that there is not a diagnosis code that maps from the source code to the target code that can identify the diagnosis. A flag does apply and is turned on.

A combination flag indicates that more than one code in the target system is required to satisfy the full equivalent meaning of a code in the source system.

Most, but not all, codes in ICD-9-CM and ICD-10-CM will have a 1 in the first position in column 3.

The third digit in the third column in Figure 9.14 is the combination flag. If the combination flag is turned on (1) from the source to the target, a combination code exists.

Now review Figure 9.14, which identifies the flags in the third column. Also review Figure 9.15, which is the GEMs text file.

FIGURE 9.15 **Illustration of Flags in GEMS**

ICD-10-CM Code	ICD-10-CM Description	ICD-9-CM Code	ICD-9-CM Description	Approximate Flag	No Map Flag	Combination Flag
R65.21	Severe sepsis with shock	995.92	Severe sepsis	1	0	1
R65.21	Severe sepsis with shock	785.52	Septic shock	1	0	1

With code R65.21 in ICD-10-CM, there is a linked code (approximate flag) and a combination code (combination flag) in the GEMs file. The scenario and choice list are the last two digits of the third column in the GEMs text files. Meanings of the third column digits are the same in both the ICD-9-CM GEMs files and the ICD-10-CM GEMs files. When a combination flag is turned on with a 1, a scenario (digit 4) and a choice list field (digit 5) will have a number other than 0. If there is a 0, a combination code does not exist.

The scenario column (Figure 9.16) is the subdivision of the hierarchy of the number of variations of a diagnosis combination included in the source system code, which is identified with a number "1," and the choice list, which is the possible target system codes that combined are one valid expression of a scenario and is identified with a number "2" in their respective columns.

The last column of the GEMs file is the choice list. For instance, if a combination code does not exist, and there is a one-to-one mapping relationship between the source code and target code, the digit is 0. If a combination code exists, there will either be a 1 or 2 in the column as follows:

- No combination codes exist; last digit in the choice column is 0
- Combination code exists with only one combination choice; last digit in the choice list is 1
- Combination code exists and more than one code-combination exists; last digit in the choice list is 2.

Review code mapping of R65.21 again before reviewing Figure 9.16.

FIGURE 9.16 **Excerpt From GEMs File, ICD-10-CM to ICD-9-CM**

| R6521 | 99592 | 1011**1** |
| R6521 | 78552 | 1011**2** |

Figure 9.16 identifies that code R65.21 has a "1," which appears as the fourth digit, indicating that for a patient with severe sepsis and shock, mapping with R65.21 requires two codes in ICD-9-CM.

FIGURE 9.17 **Example of GEMs Text File**

ICD-10-CM Code	ICD-10-CM Description	ICD-9-CM Code	ICD-9-CM Description	Approximate Flag	No Map Flag	Combination Flag	Scenario	Choice List
R65.21	Severe sepsis with shock	995.92	Severe sepsis	1	0	1	1	1
R65.21	Severe sepsis with shock	785.52	Septic shock	1	0	1	1	2

In Figure 9.16, code 995.92 can map only to R65.21, because there is not a code in ICD-10-CM to cover sepsis only. However, R65.21 maps to 995.92 and 785.52.

In a practice, it would not be necessary to map every code in ICD-9-CM to ICD-10-CM and map every code in ICD-10-CM back to ICD-9-CM. As stated earlier, software vendors will typically map ICD-9-CM to ICD-10-CM and ICD-10-CM back to ICD-9-CM. However, each practice will need to crosswalk and map Superbills if the practitioner decides to continue to use this tool for tracking procedures and services.

Health plans and/or hospitals might map all of ICD-9-CM and ICD-10-CM because their ICD-9-CM code use is more extensive. However, it is still important for each practice to map and crosswalk between the two coding systems prior to ICD-10-CM implementation, if necessary.

Here are some key steps to follow in the use of GEMs files:

1   It is best to use a database when using the GEMs text files.

2   Make sure the person using the system understands coding and crosswalks.

3   Obtain the GEMs files from the Centers for Medicare & Medicaid Services Web site at www.cms.hhs.gov/ICD10. The files are in a zip format, and the user will need to save the files to the computer's hard drive.

4   Once the files are unzipped, review the guidelines for using the GEMs. The guidelines may need to be read several times for understanding of the methodology.

5   After reading the instructions, pull down the ICD-9-CM text files from the CDC Web site mentioned earlier, which will be useful for ICD-9-CM descriptors in the GEMs files.

6   Begin mapping the files from ICD-9-CM (source) to ICD-10-CM (target).

7   After completing the forward mapping, do the reverse mapping. Map from ICD-10-CM (source) to ICD-9-CM (target).

> **INFORMATION TECHNOLOGY SYSTEM TIP**
>
> Even though the information technology systems vendor or practice staff will most likely do the crosswalking and mapping to ICD-10-CM, understanding the relationship between the ICD-9-CM and ICD-10-CM code sets will be beneficial for the practice. In addition, the practice will need to understand these cross-walks in order to convert each ICD-9-CM code on the Superbill to its equivalent ICD-10-CM code or codes.

Summary

It is important for any practice, small or large, to review and understand the GEMs files to understand the relationship between mapping from the ICD-9-CM codes to the ICD-10-CM codes and from the ICD-10-CM codes back to the ICD-9-CM codes. As ICD-10-CM moves ahead, vendors may be available to map and crosswalk within information technology systems, but everyone needs to understand the crosswalk between both coding systems by mapping the most common diagnoses performed in the practice. This might help the practice decide whether the continued use of Superbills is beneficial or is cumbersome and should be replaced.

Resources

ICD-10-CM General Equivalence Mappings Files and Instructions. Available online at www.cms.hhs.gov/ICD10/02m_2009_ICD_10_CM.asp#TopOfPage.

Centers for Disease Control and Prevention. National Center for Health Statistics. *Classifications of Diseases and Functioning & Disability*. Available online at www.cdc.gov/nchs/icd9.htm#RTF.

End-of-Chapter Questions

1   The acronym *GEMs* stands for: _____.

2   The core classification in ICD-10-CM is:

   _____.

3   Explain how the GEMs files are formatted.

   _____

4   In the GEMs, there are flags that identify combination codes that map

   from the _____ to the _____ of the table.

5   Where can a practice obtain the GEMs files?

   _____

APPENDIX A

End-of-Chapter Questions With Answers

Chapter 1

1   ICD-10-CM will have **up to seven character extensions**.

2   *WHO* stands for **World Health Organization.**

3   ICD-10-CM is currently used in the United States for **coding and classifying mortality data from death certificates**.

4   The ICD-10-CM format is:
    b   **alphanumeric.**

5   ICD-10-CM is published in a **three** volume set.

Chapter 2

1   The clinical modification of ICD-9 (ICD-9-CM, Volumes 1 and 2), which is used today for reporting morbidities, was adopted in what year?
    1978

2   The organization that conducted the impact analysis study for migration to ICD-10 is **the RAND Science and Technology Policy Institute**.

3   For physician providers, the realized benefits of ICD-10-CM include:
    a   **more precise documentation of clinical care.**
    b   **more accurate coding.**
    c   **the contribution to health care quality improvement initiatives.**

Chapter 3

1   According to the RAND study, there are three types of costs to providers. What are these potential costs?
    a   **cost of training physicians, coders, billers, and others**
    b   **cost of lost productivity**
    c   **cost of system changes**

2   Productivity might be impacted with ICD-10-CM implementation. Which three key areas might cause short-term productivity issues?
    a   **queries from coders to clarify documentation in the medical record**
    b   **increased billing inquiries by payers**
    c   **increased number of adjustments and pending or suspended claims**

3   What two significant challenges might the United States have with ICD-10-CM implementation?
    a   **shortage of health care professionals**
    b   **resistance to change**

4 Why is diagnosis coding so important to the physician submitting claims for payment?

> **It supports medical necessity for services reported.**

5 The American Health Information Management Association field testing study identified some problems with ICD-10-CM. What were they?

> a **nonspecific codes**
>
> b **unclear guidelines and instructions**
>
> c **lack of coding tools**
>
> d **requirement for training**
>
> e **reduced productivity during and after implementation**

Chapter 4

1 Name the five recommended steps for ICD-10-CM implementation in the practice.

> a **creation of a committee**
>
> b **budget planning**
>
> c **creation of a timeline**
>
> d **identification of training needs**
>
> e **information management system upgrades and review**

2 For budgeting, what is the average dollar amount that a practice might spend on system upgrades?

> **between $4,000 and $10,000, depending on systems used in the practice**

3 When a budget is created, what other expenditures besides system upgrades need to be considered?

> **consulting services, review of documentation, training, and overtime**

4 Why is a documentation review/audit beneficial for preparation for ICD-10-CM implementation?

> **to validate or ensure that the practitioner is documenting to the level of specificity required in ICD-10-CM**

5 List the six types of training media available today.

> a **classroom**
>
> b **seminars**
>
> c **courses**
>
> d **distance learning or webinars**
>
> e **self-study**
>
> f **boot camps**

Chapter 5

1   The Alphabetic Index in ICD-10-CM is divided into what two parts?
    Index to Disease and Injury and Index to External Causes of Injury

2   Chapters are further divided into **subchapters or blocks**.

3   ICD-10-CM uses dummy placeholders defined by the letter **x**.

4   The *Excludes 1* convention indicates **that the code is excluded and should never be used at the same time as the code above the Excludes 1 note and that the two conditions cannot occur together**.

5   The *Excludes 2* convention indicates **that the condition is excluded and not part of the condition, but the patient may have both conditions at the same time, and both codes may be reported together**.

Chapter 6

1   The *ICD-10-CM Official Guidelines for Coding and Reporting* are organized into which sections?
    Section 1, ICD-10-CM Conventions
    Section 2, General Coding Guidelines
    Section 3, Chapter-Specific Guidelines

2   Coding for signs or symptoms should be used only when:
    no definitive diagnosis is established at the time the patient encounter is coded. When the diagnosis is confirmed prior to coding of the encounter, the confirmed diagnosis is reported.

3   Laterality is indicated by the **final** character of the code.

4   When an encounter is for a pathological fracture due to a malignancy, what subcategory would the user reference for the diagnosis?
    subcategory M84.5

5   The subcategories for chemotherapy and radiation therapy are:
    Z51.11 Chemotherapy and Z51.0 Radiation therapy.

Chapter 7

1   In ICD-9-CM, diseases of the eye and adnexa are located with **Nervous system**, but in ICD-10-CM, the codes are located in Chapter **7**.

2   Codes for hypertensive heart disease in ICD-10-CM are found in what categories?
    I10 to I15

3   How is secondary hypertension reported in ICD-10-CM?
    Two codes are required—one code to identify the underlying etiology and one code from I15 to report the hypertension.

4   If a patient has multiple complications of Crohn's disease, **multiple codes** may be reported from **K50 or K51** for each complication.

5   When coma is being coded in ICD-10-CM, what must be used in conjunction with the coma codes for brain injuries or the sequelae of cerebrovascular accidents?
    Glasgow coma scale

Chapter 8

1   In the Table of Drugs and Chemicals, the poisoning codes for undetermined intent should be used only when **specific documentation in the record indicates the intent could not be determined**.

2   How are poisoning codes sequenced?
    Code first the poisoning code from category T36 to T50, then code the nature of the poisoning by the codes that specified the poisoning (patient's condition).

3   The three common seventh character extensions are:
    A initial encounter
    B subsequent encounter
    C sequela.

4   How should spinal cord injuries be reported, based on the ICD-10-CM guidelines?
    For each section of spinal cord injury, code for the highest level of injury for that section of the cord. If a patient has a cord injury at more than one section of the cord, report the code for the highest level of injury for each section.

5   Burn codes are classified by **site**, **depth**, and **degree (first, second, and third degree).**

Chapter 9

1   The acronym *GEMs* stands for **General Equivalence Mappings**.

2   The core classification in ICD-10-CM is the **three-character code**.

3   Explain how the GEMs files are formatted.
    GEMs files are flat text files in which each file contains a list of code pairs that identify the correspondence between a source system code and a target system code.

4   In the GEMs, there are flags that identify combination codes that map from the **source** to the **target** of the table.

5   Where can a practice obtain the GEMs files?

> **GEMs files can be obtained from the Centers for Medicare & Medicaid Services Web site at www.cms.hhs.gov/ICD10/02m_2009_ ICD_10_CM.asp#TopOfPage**

ICD-10-CM Terminology

ICD-10-CM Terminology

AAPC: American Academy of Professional Coders. National organization dedicated to promoting professional standards and recognition for professional coders and certification for outpatient hospital, physician practices, and payers.

AHIMA: American Health Information Management Association. National organization promoting the art and science of medical record management and improving the quality of comprehensive health information and certification.

Alphabetic Index: The ICD-10-CM Index to Diseases and Injuries is the alphabetical list of disease/injury terms in ICD-10-CM.

American Medical Association: The largest US professional association of physicians and publisher of Current Procedural Terminology®, Fourth Edition (CPT-4).

And: When the term *and* is used in a narrative statement, it represents and/or.

Base: The classification system from which all codes are matched to selected codes from another classification system. The base system acts as the starting point from which codes are translated from one classification system to another.

Brackets: Brackets are used in the Tabular List to enclose synonyms, alternative wording or explanatory phrases. Brackets are used in the Alphabetic Index to identify manifestation codes (see **Code first/Use additional code** convention).

Centers for Medicare & Medicaid Services (CMS): CMS is a federal agency within the US Department of Health and Human Services. Programs for which CMS is responsible include Medicare, Medicaid, and the Health Insurance Portability and Accountability Act (HIPAA).

CMS-1500 claim form: The standard insurance claim form used to report outpatient service to insurance carriers.

Code also note: A *code also* note instructs that two codes may be required to fully describe a condition, but the sequencing of the two codes depends on the severity of the conditions and the reason for the encounter. See subcategory H05.32 for an example of this convention.

Code first/use additional code note (etiology/manifestation paired codes): ICD-10-CM coding convention used when conditions have both an underlying etiology and multiple body system manifestations due to the underlying etiology. The underlying condition is sequenced first, followed by the manifestation. Wherever such a combination exists there is a *use additional code* note at the etiology code and a *code first* note at the manifestation code. These instructional notes indicate the proper sequencing order of the codes—etiology followed by manifestation.

Coder: A professional who translates documentation, written diagnostics, and procedures into numeric and alphanumeric codes.

Coding: Transferring a narrative description of diseases, injuries, and procedures into a numeric designation.

Colon: Used in the Tabular List after an incomplete term that needs one or more of the modifiers following the colon to make it assignable to a given category.

Comorbidity: An ongoing condition that exists along with the condition(s) for which the patient is receiving treatment.

Complication: Disease or condition arising during the course of, or as a result of, another disease-modifying medical treatment or outcome.

Conversion: The single reference system code that best matches a single base system code. Each conversion should indicate a useful one-to-one match for each base code, for users interested in broad category "fits" that allow every base code to be represented by a single reference code. In general, a given crosswalk is likely to lead a user toward extraneous data, but a given conversion is likely to lead toward some type of data or information loss at the code level.

Crosswalk: The complete set of reference system codes that match a single base system code. In general, crosswalks should lead a user toward where to find all potential data matches for a base code but (at the same time) may also lead toward extraneous data, because of differences in the (inclusion and exclusion) classification structure between the base and reference codes involved.

Current Procedural Terminology (CPT®) Codes: CPT codes are a listing of descriptive terms and identifying codes for reporting medical services and procedures. The purpose of CPT is to provide a uniform language that accurately describes medical, surgical, and diagnostic services. CPT is a trademark of the American Medical Association.

Department of Health and Human Services (DHHS): DHHS is the US government's principal agency for protecting the health of all Americans and providing essential human services, especially for those who are least able to help themselves. The Department includes more than 300 programs, covering a wide spectrum of activities including health and social science research, Medicare and Medicaid, and medical preparedness for emergencies, including potential terrorism.

Diagnosis-related groups (DRGs): The DRGs work by grouping ICD codes into a more manageable number of meaningful patient categories (approximately 500 in 2003). They are grouped into cohorts based on clinical and resource use characteristics and demographic data.

Documentation: Chronological detailed recording of pertinent facts and observations about a patient's health recorded in the medical chart and associated reports.

Electronic health record (EHR): An electronic information system framework that captures data at the point of care, integrates data from multiple sources, and supports real-time caregiver decision making.

Etiology: The cause of disease.

Excludes note: The ICD-10-CM has two types of excludes notes. Each note has a different definition, but they are similar in that they indicate that codes excluded from each other are independent of each other.

- **Excludes1:** A type one excludes note is a pure excludes. It means "not coded here." An *Excludes1* note indicates that the code excluded should never be used at the same time as the code above the *Excludes1* note. An *Excludes1* is used when two conditions cannot occur together, such as a congenital form and an acquired form of the same condition.
- **Excludes2:** A type two excludes note represents "not included here." An *Excludes2* note indicates that the condition excluded is not part of the condition represented by the code, but a patient may have both conditions at the same time. When an *Excludes2* note appears under a code, it is acceptable to use both the code and the excluded code together if both conditions exist.

Includes note: The word *includes* appears immediately under certain categories to further define, or give examples of, the content of the category.

Inclusion term: Lists of terms are included under some codes. These terms are some of the conditions for which that code number is to be used. The terms may be synonyms of the code title, or, in the case of *other specified* codes, the terms are a list of some of the various conditions assigned to that code. The inclusion terms are not necessarily exhaustive. Additional terms found only in the Alphabetic Index may also be assigned to a code.

Inpatient: A patient who is admitted to a hospital for a period of time.

Insured: An individual or organization protected by insurance in case of loss under the specific terms of the insurance policy.

International Classification of Diseases (ICD): Classification system used to group clinical conditions and procedures into manageable categories for external reporting purposes, including reimbursement for health care services as well as statistical data analysis, such as epidemiological analysis or trending of disease incidence.

- **ICD-9-CM:** International Classification of Diseases, Ninth Revision, Clinical Modification (a US version of ICD-9 developed by the World Health Organization). ICD-9-CM is divided into three volumes. Volumes I and II relate to diagnosis classification, whereas Volume III relates to inpatient procedure classification. ICD-9-CM has approximately 13,000 diagnosis codes with 855 code categories (3-5 alphanumeric characters) and 4,000 procedure codes (3-4 numeric characters).
- **ICD-10-CM:** International Classification of Diseases, Tenth Revision, Clinical Modification (a US version of ICD-10 developed by the World Health Organization). ICD-10-CM has approximately 120,000 codes with 2,033 code categories (3-7 alphanumeric characters).

Late effect: Inactive residual effect or condition produced after the acute phase of an injury or illness has ended.

Mapping: The process of linking content from one terminology or classification scheme to another.

Match: The set of codes from one classification system that are equivalent or nearest-to-equivalent to a code from another classification system constitute a match. A complete set of matches provides a means for translating codes from one classification system to another. Crosswalks and conversions (defined earlier) are different types of matches.

Medical necessity: Specific diagnostic requirements for a specific service to indicate medical need.

Morbidity: A diseased state, often used in the context of a *morbidity rate* (ie, the rate of disease or proportion of diseased people in a population). In common clinical usage, any disease state, including diagnosis and complications, is referred to as morbidity.

National Center for Health Statistics (NCHS): NCHS serves as the World Health Organization Collaborating Center for the Family of International Classifications for North America and in this capacity is responsible for coordination of all official disease classification activities in the United States relating to the ICD and its use, interpretation, and periodic revision.

National Committee on Vital and Health Statistics (NCVHS): The NCVHS serves as the statutory public advisory body to the Secretary of Health and Human Services in the area of health data and statistics. In that capacity, the Committee provides advice and assistance to the Department and serves as a forum for interaction with interested private sector groups on a variety of key health data issues.

Not elsewhere classifiable (NEC): NEC represents *other specified* in ICD-10-CM. An index entry that states NEC directs the coder to an *other specified* code in the Tabular List (see **Inclusion terms**).

Not otherwise specified (NOS): Codes in the Tabular List with *unspecified* in the title (usually a code with a fourth or sixth character 9 and fifth character 0) are used when the information in the medical record is insufficient to assign a more specific code. The abbreviation NOS in the Tabular List is the equivalent of unspecified.

Outpatient: A person who encounters health services in a physician's office, hospital clinic, or the office of other providers of health care services.

Parentheses: Parentheses are used in both the Alphabetic Index and Tabular List to enclose supplementary words that may be present or absent in the statement of a disease or procedure without affecting the code number to which it is assigned. The terms within the parentheses are referred to as *nonessential modifiers*.

Poisoning: An adverse medical state caused by an overdose of medication, the prescription and use of a medicinal substance prescribed in error, or a drug mistakenly ingested or applied.

Principal/first listed diagnosis: The condition considered to be the major health problem for the patient, always listed and coded first on the claim form.

Provider: A physician or other supplier of medical services or equipment.

The RAND Corporation: The RAND Corporation is a nonprofit research organization providing objective analysis and effective solutions that address the challenges facing the public and private sectors around the world.

See: Directs the user to a more specific term in ICD-10-CM under which the correct code can be found.

See also: Indicates that additional information is available in ICD-10-CM that may provide an additional diagnostic code.

See category: Indicates that the user should review the category specified before assigning a code in ICD-10-CM.

SNOMED-CT: A comprehensive, multilingual, controlled clinical terminology or common reference terminology containing more than 300,000 concepts. SNOMED-CT is designed to support the EHR, enabling the development of richer computer-aided clinical decision support systems, critical care monitoring, facilitating communication among clinicians, use in clinical trials and computerized physician order entry systems, and improving the quality of data available for research and measurement of clinical outcomes.

Tabular List: The numerical listing of diseases found in ICD-9-CM, known as Volume 1 of ICD-10-CM.

Unspecified nature: A description for a neoplasm when the histology or nature of the tumor has not yet been determined.

Volume 1 of ICD-10-CM: The tabular list of diseases in ICD-10-CM listed in numerical order by chapter.

Volume 2 of ICD-10-CM: The alphabetical index to Volume 1 that lists diseases and etiology.

With/without note: When *with* and *without* are the two options for the final character of a set of codes, the default is always *without*. For five-character codes, a 0 as the fifth position character represents *without*, and 1 represents *with*. For six-character codes, the sixth position character 1 represents *with*, and 9 represents *without*.

APPENDIX C

Web Sites and Resource Materials

Valuable Web Sites

General

Office of the Inspector General (Useful for gaining coding compliance information)	www.oig.hhs.gov/authorities/docs/physician.pdf
Acronym Finder (Useful for referencing definitions of acronyms)	www.acronymfinder.com/
American Academy of Professional Coders, ICD-10	www.aapc.com/ICD-0/index.aspx
American College of Healthcare Executives	www.ache.org
American College of Legal Medicine	www.aclm.org
American College of Surgeons	www.facs.org
American Health Information Management Association, ICD-10	www.ahima.org/icd10/index.asp
American Medical Association	www.ama-assn.org
Health Care Compliance Association	www.hcca-info.org
Health Information Media Products (Useful for obtaining reference materials)	www.adam.com
Healthcare Financial Management Association	www.hfma.org
Medical Association of Billers	www.physicianswebsites.com
Medical Group Management Association	www.mgma.com/
Online Medicare coding/billing training	www.cms.hhs.gov/MLNGenInfo/
RAND Technical Report	www.rand.org/pubs/technical_reports/TR132
The Free Dictionary	www.acronyms.thefreedictionary.com/ICD-10-CM
US National Library of Medicine	www.nlm.nih.gov/
Web MD	www.webmd.com/
Workgroup for Electronic Data Interchange	www.wedi.org/
World Health Organization	www.who.int/en/

Government

Agency for Healthcare Research and Quality	www.ahrq.gov/
Centers for Disease Control and Prevention/ US Department of Health and Human Services, ICD-10-CM	www.cdc.gov/nchs/about/major/dvs/icd10des.htm
Centers for Medicare and Medicaid Services (CMS)	www.cms.hhs.gov/ICD10
Code of Federal Regulations	www.gpoaccess.gov/cfr/index.html
Federal Register	www.gpoaccess.gov/fr/index.html
Fedworld Information Network/US Department of Commerce	www.fedworld.gov
Joint Commission (The)	www.jointcommission.org/
National Committee for Quality Assurance (The)	www.ncqa.org
National Committee on Vital and Health Statistics	www.ncvhs.hhs.gov/
National Health Information Center/US Department of Health & Human Services	www.healthfinder.gov
National Institutes of Health/US Department of Health and Human Services	www.nih.gov
Office for Civil Rights—HIPAA/Medical Privacy—National Standards to Protect the Privacy of Personal Health Information	www.hhs.gov/ocr/office/index.html
Office of Inspector General (OIG)	oig.hhs.gov/
US Government Printing Office	www.access.gpo.gov

Medicolegal

American Health Lawyers Association   www.healthlawyers.org

MediRegs (search engine for managing health   www.mediregs.com/index.html
care compliance information)

National Health Care Anti-Fraud Association   www.nhcaa.org

Resource Materials

Centers for Medicare & Medicaid Services   www.cms.hhs.org/ICD-10

Coding Clinic, American Hospital Association   www.aha.org

ICD-10-CM Draft Guidelines; Alphabetic Index; www.cms.hhs.org/ICD-10
Tabular List; Table of Drugs and Chemicals;
GEMs files

Index